This book is dedicated to my wife Courtney and five children without whom this book would not be possible.

© Copyright 2021 by Adam Voydik – All rights reserved.

It is illegal to reproduce, duplicate or transmit any part of this document in either electronic means or printed format. Recording of this publication is strictly prohibited.

Introduction

Congratulations on purchasing ACLS Fundamentals a Study Guide to Pass the First Time. This book details Advanced Cardiovascular Life Support (ACLS) content per the current 2020 American Heart Association (AHA) emergency cardiovascular care (ECC) guidelines. This book is not endorsed by the AHA and must not be construed as a primary reference document for ECC guidelines.

ACLS ECC guidelines direct adult-oriented patient care, whereby ACLS providers administer medications, navigate treatment algorithms, interpret electrocardiograms (ECG), and communicate effectively with team members. ACLS Fundamentals breaks down the core concepts required to pass the ACLS Provider course. The chapters of this book build on one another to reinforce memory retention.

The ACLS Provider Manual numbers 202 pages and covers a great deal of information. ACLS Fundamentals ideally summarizes the information within the ACLS Provider Manual and familiarizes the reader with ACLS in a concise manner. All AHA courses are **OPEN RESOURCE** and allow for the use of the provider manual, algorithm sheets, and notes.

This book is written as a quick read utilizing simple diagrams, checks on learning, a pre and posttest, mnemonics, and video links to ensure content mastery. Attempt the ACLS course shortly after reading this book to maximize your success. EMskillz, LLC provides regular course offerings for Basic Life Support (BLS), Advanced Cardiovascular Life Support (ACLS), and Pediatric Advanced Life Support (PALS).

The author of this book instructs ACLS per the AHA's published curriculum, is a Certified Flight Paramedic and Nationally Registered Paramedic with 15 years of experience working in the critical care setting. The proceeding content mirrors the author's teaching style, which has aided numerous students to pass the AHA's ACLS Provider course on their first attempt. Visit emskillz.com to see our available course offerings. Feel free to contact the author about any questions or concerns that you may have by emailing training@emskillz.com. Thank you again and happy reading.

How to Read this Book

ACLS students will be evaluated on their performance of adult BLS, airway management, and a high-performance team activity (megacode). ACLS is a broad subject covering a variety of topics. To reinforce key concepts the following memory retention methods are utilized. When you see the following items recognize that this information is vitally important.

Warning signs are found throughout the chapters to catch your attention to outline critical performance steps.

QR codes accompanied by a video title direct you to EMskillz.com/emflix, where deeper explanations of concepts not easily explained by words and pictures alone are provided.

Checks on learning are found throughout each chapter and cover material from the preceding sections.

Pearls of wisdom are found at the beginning of each subject area. The items within these blocks comprise testable information.

Table of Contents

Pretest.. 5
Chapter 1: The Systematic Approach................................... 16
Chapter 2: Basic Life Support..18
Chapter 3: Cardiovascular System Review........................... 21
Chapter 4: ECG Interpretation...23
Chapter 5: Algorithms...29
Chapter 6: Airway Management.. 46
Chapter 7: High Performance Teams.................................... 49
Chapter 8: The Megacode Overview...................................... 51
Posttest...60
Conclusion.. 71
References..72
Pretest and Posttest Answer Keys... 73
Check on Learning Answers... 74
Emergency Cardiovascular Care Data Sheet........................ 79
ECG Analysis Tool..78

Pretest

1. How much aspirin would a telecommunicator direct a rescuer to administer for someone complaining of chest pain?
    a. 81 mg
    b. 324 mg
    c. 325 mg
    d. 162 mg - 325 mg

2. A patient experiencing chest pain with a history of coronary artery stent placement is most likely suffering from what?
    a. Acute stroke
    b. Acute coronary syndrome
    c. Tension pneumothorax
    d. Gallstones

3. Identify this rhythm.

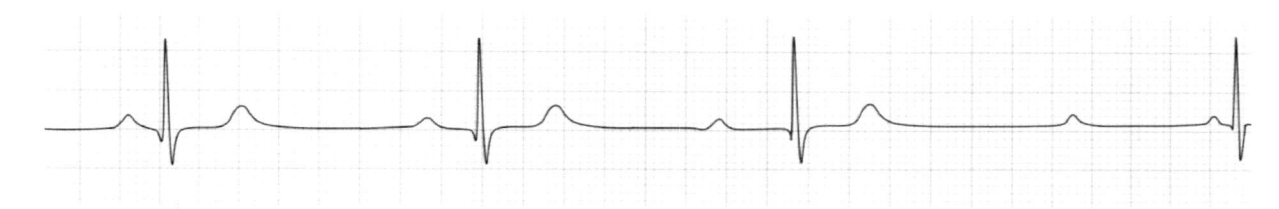

    a. Sinus bradycardia
    b. Second degree AV block type I
    c. Second degree AV block type II
    d. Third degree AV block

4. A patient in the emergency department waiting room collapses and remains unconscious, what is the next appropriate step a rescuer should take?
    a. Acquire a 12-lead ECG
    b. Perform a BLS assessment
    c. Begin CPR
    d. Provide rescue breaths

5.) Placement of an advanced airway should be confirmed by way of method?

   a. Chest x-ray

   b. Arterial blood gas

   c. Continuous waveform capnography

   d. Positive pressure ventilations

The following scenario applies to questions 6-10

Scenario: A 59-year-old man is being treated for chest pain and he appears diaphoretic, in obvious discomfort, and lightheaded. He has no prior medical history of cardiovascular disease. The 12-lead ECG reveals the rhythm below, which suddenly converts to ventricular fibrillation.

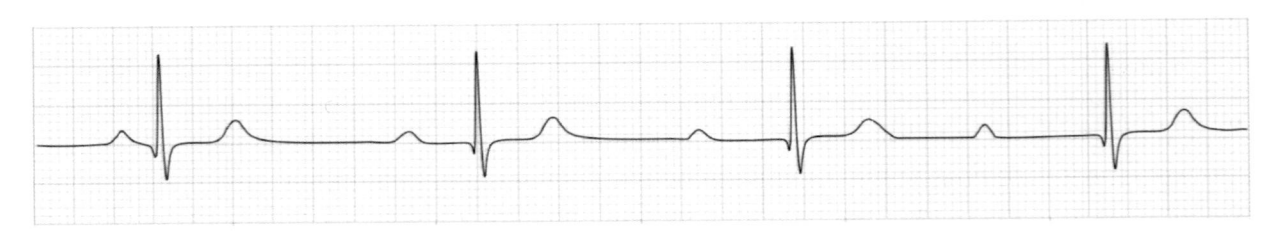

6. Identify the above rhythm.

   a. Wolff-Parkinson-White syndrome

   b. First degree AV block

   c. Second degree AV block type II

   d. Third degree AV block

7. What is the next most appropriate action to care for this patient?

   a. Place an advanced airway

   b. Perform defibrillation

   c. Perform synchronized cardioversion

   d. Perform transcutaneous pacing

8. Which medication should be administered first per the algorithm?

   a. Dopamine 2 mcg - 10 mcg/min

   b. Adenosine 12 mg

   c. Epinephrine 1 mg

   d. Amiodarone 300 mg

9. Despite the medication provided above the patient remains in ventricular fibrillation. Which medication should be provided next?
    a. Amiodarone 300 mg
    b. Epinephrine 1 mg
    c. Magnesium Sulfate 4 gm
    d. Epinephrine 2 mcg - 10 mcg/min

10. If the patient had not gone into ventricular fibrillation, what would have been the appropriate treatment?
    a. Synchronized cardioversion
    b. Vagal maneuvers
    c. Transcutaneous pacing
    d. Defibrillation

11. You are transporting a suspected stroke patient, what course of action takes priority upon arrival to the medical facility?
    a. Fibrinolytic therapy
    b. 12-lead ECG
    c. Pericardiocentesis
    d. CT scan

12. Patients suspected of having an acute coronary syndrome should be taken to which type of facility?
    a. Coronary reperfusion-capable facility
    b. Dialysis-capable facility
    c. A stroke center
    d. A level III trauma center

13. You are treating a suspected stroke patient who has a normal CT scan and has been experiencing symptoms for the last five hours, what is the next step in treatment?
    a. Request an MRI to confirm the CT scan
    b. Administer Fibrinolytic Therapy Immediately
    c. Refer patient for mechanical thrombectomy
    d. The patient requires no interventions

14. You are treating a patient with the below rhythm and is pulseless, what is the appropriate treatment?

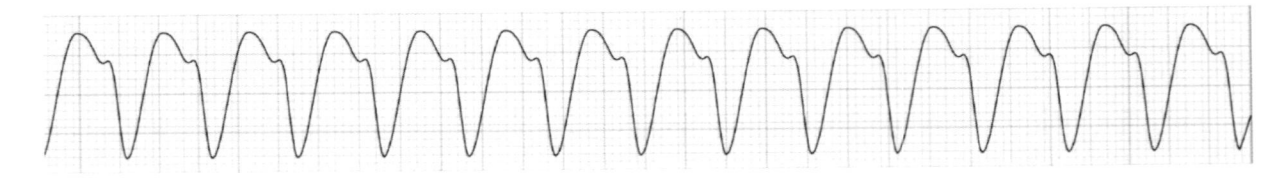

   a. Perform synchronized cardioversion
   b. Administer adenosine 6 mg
   c. Administer epinephrine 1 mg
   d. Perform defibrillation

15. Which action should immediately follow a defibrillation attempt?
   a. High-quality CPR
   b. Pulse/rhythm check
   c. Medication administration
   d. Another defibrillation if first attempt failed to resolve the rhythm

16. You notice a colleague performing shallow chest compressions, how should you address this?
   a. Wait until the end of the resuscitation
   b. Immediately take over chest compressions
   c. Say, "your compressions are wrong."
   d. Say, "ensure your compressions are 2 inches deep allowing for recoil."

17. The monitor displays a PETCO2 reading of 6 mmHg, what does this indicate?
   a. The patient is being hyperventilated
   b. Chest compressions are ineffective
   c. The patient is being hypoventilated
   d. The patient is developing a tension pneumothorax

18. You enter your patient's room, and they appear to be unconscious, but you hear them gasping, what action should be performed?
   a. Check the pulse oximeter reading
   b. Begin high-quality CPR the gasping is not normal breathing
   c. The gasping is normal breathing, and the patient does not require care
   d. Check the patient's blood glucose

19. Identify this rhythm

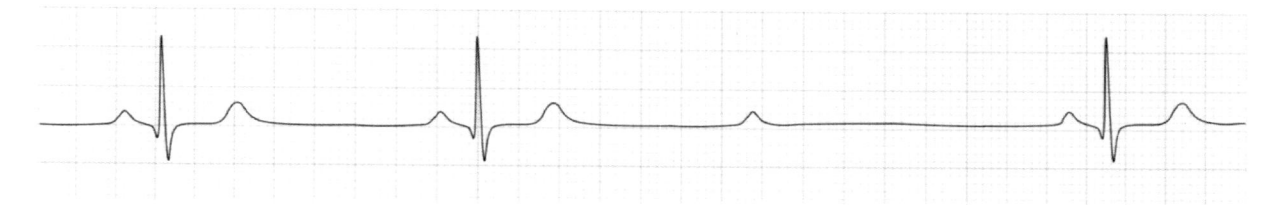

a. First degree AV block
b. Second degree AV block Type I
c. Second degree AV block Type II
d. Third degree AV block

20. You are treating a patient who just achieved ROSC but is unable to follow your commands, what treatment should be considered?

a. 2 L fluid bolus
b. Targeted temperature management
c. Administer epinephrine 5 mcg/min drip
d. Provide positive pressure ventilation 1 breath every 10 seconds

21. How is an OPA properly measured?

a. From the corner of the nose to the earlobe
b. From the corner of the mouth to the Adam's apple
c. From the corner of the mouth to the corner of the jaw
d. Sizes are universal, and measurement is not required

22. Targeted temperature management is provided at what temperature range?

a. 30°C-34°C
b. 31°C-35°C
c. 32°C-36°C
d. 33°C-37°C

23. How long should targeted temperature management be administered?

a. 12 hours
b. 24 hours
c. 36 hours
d. 48 hours

24. Increase chest compression fraction by performing what actions?
    a. Administer breaths while chest compressions are ongoing
    b. Administer medications while chest compressions are ongoing
    c. Switch compressors every two minutes
    d. Charge the defibrillator prior to the 2-minute mark

25. What reading provides insight into compression effectiveness?
    a. A palpable femoral pulse
    b. PETCO2 reading of at least 10 mmHg
    c. Pulse oxygen saturation
    d. Core body temperature

26. What is the purpose of having a CPR Coach?
    a. Ensure high-quality CPR is being performed
    b. Facilitate knowledge sharing
    c. To tell the team leader when he/she is wrong
    d. To perform defibrillation

27. What is the first medical intervention to balloon time for a STEMI patient?
    a. 30 minutes
    b. 60 minutes
    c. 90 minutes
    d. 120 minutes

28. What is the proper closed loop response for an order of amiodarone 300 mg?
    a. "Ok, got it.'
    b. "I have an order for amiodarone 300 mg."
    c. "Is that really what you want to give?"
    d. "I don't think that is correct."

29. How often should a breath be provided while performing rescue breaths?
    a. 1 breath every 2-3 seconds
    b. 1 breath every 5 seconds
    c. 1 breath every 6 seconds
    d. 1 breath every 10 seconds

30. A patient with a pulse and hypotension presents with the below rhythm, what action should be performed?

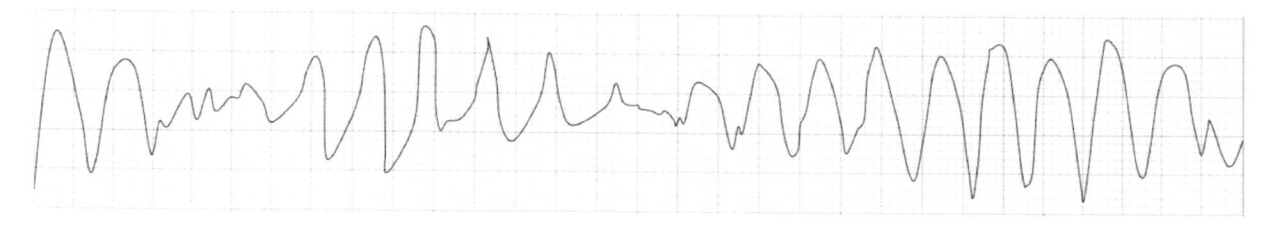

a. Defibrillation
b. Synchronized cardioversion
c. Amiodarone 150 mg
d. Dopamine 5 mg - 20 mg/kg/min infusion

31. Avoid excessive ventilation because it causes what?
a. Optimal oxygenation
b. Diminished cardiac output
c. Improved circulation
d. Decreased thoracic pressures

The following scenario applies to questions 32-40

Scenario: A 71-year-old patient was brought into the emergency department complaining of chest tightness, nausea, and dizziness. He explains that he had a heart attack two years ago.

32. What is the first and most important action to be taken?
a. 12-lead ECG
b. Cardiac panel
c. ABG
d. Blood glucose

33. The monitor reveals the below rhythm, identify this rhythm.

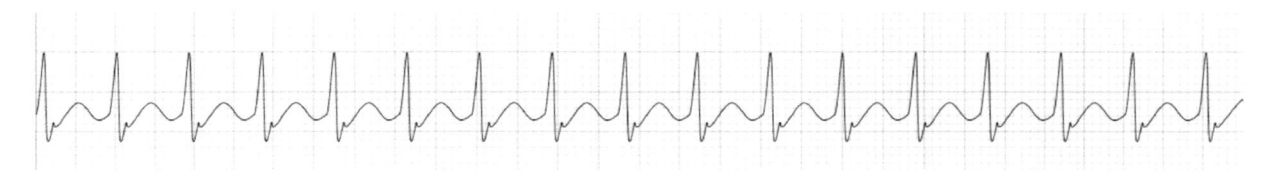

a. Atrial fibrillation

b. Atrial flutter

c. Sinus tachycardia

d. Supraventricular tachycardia

34. Given the patient's presentation and the above rhythm, what algorithm would be used to treat this patient?

    a. Cardiac arrest VF/pVT

    b. Adult tachycardia with a pulse

    c. Bradycardia

    d. Cardiac arrest PEA/Asystole

35. The patient's blood pressure is 84/68 mmHg. What is the most appropriate treatment for this patient?

    a. Vagal maneuvers

    b. Adenosine 6 mg

    c. Adenosine 12 mg

    d. Synchronized cardioversion

36. Despite the action above the patient's rhythm remains the same and the patient remains conscious. What is the next appropriate treatment?

    a. Vagal maneuvers

    b. Adenosine 6 mg

    c. Adenosine 12 mg

    d. Synchronized cardioversion

37. The patient goes unconscious, and the below rhythm presents on the monitor. What algorithm should the patient be treated under?

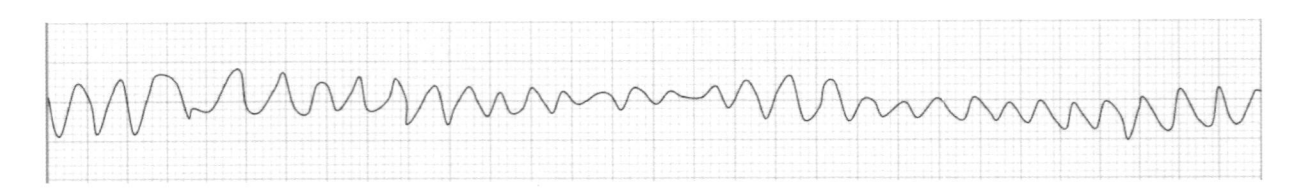

a. Cardiac arrest VF/pVT

b. Adult tachycardia with a pulse

c. Bradycardia

d. Cardiac arrest PEA/Asystole

38. Despite 2 defibrillation attempts, and epinephrine 1 mg the patient's condition does not improve. What medication should be given following the next defibrillation attempt?

　　a. Lidocaine 1.5 mg IV push

　　b. Atropine 1 mg IV push

　　c. Beta blocker

　　d. Adenosine 300 mg

39. The patient has a ROSC and remains unconscious. What should his minimum systolic blood pressure be?

　　a. 80 mmHg

　　b. 90 mmHg

　　c. 94 mmHg

　　d. 100 mmHg

40. Due to your patient being unconscious and unable to maintain an adequate ventilatory rate, what action takes priority?

　　a. Lab values

　　b. Chest x-ray

　　c. Oxygen administration

　　d. Advanced airway management

41. For a suspected stroke patient to receive fibrinolytic therapy they must have a symptom onset to needle time of what?

　　a. 1 hour

　　b. 1.5 hours

　　c. 2 hours

　　d. 3 hours

42. Which symptom indicates cardiac arrest

   a. Agonal gasps

   b. Erythema

   c. Ecchymosis

   d. Weak and thready pulse

43. If you notice that the team leader is becoming fixated on a particular course of action or therapy, what high-performance team dynamic should be utilized?

   a. Constructive intervention

   b. Knowledge sharing

   c. Establishing clear roles and responsibilities

   d. Identifying limitations

44. You are caring for a patient whose oxygen saturation is 88% on room air, what is an indicated treatment?

   a. Oxygen via non-rebreather mask

   b. Positive pressure ventilation

   c. Patient positioning

   d. Advanced airway management

45. Your patient complained of a fluttering feeling in their chest but denies any past medical history of cardiovascular disease. The below rhythm is seen on the monitor, your patient's blood pressure is 100/84, and does not appear to be in distress. What should your first course of action be?

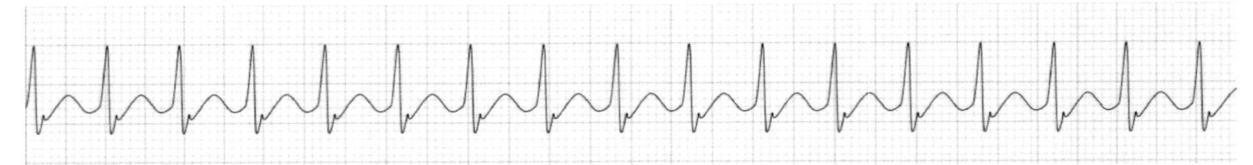

   a. Expert consultation

   b. Adenosine 6 mg

   c. Synchronized cardioversion

   d. Vagal maneuvers

46. What is the purpose of Medical Emergency Teams (MET) and Rapid Response Teams (RRT)?
   a. Provide guidance to resuscitation teams
   b. Improve patient outcomes by identifying clinical deterioration early
   c. Augment surgical teams in the event the patient enters cardiac arrest
   d. Facilitate patient transfers between EMS and the receiving hospital

47. A 53-year-old male is receiving chest compressions and at the two-minute mark remains pulseless, but this rhythm appears on the monitor. What should occur next?

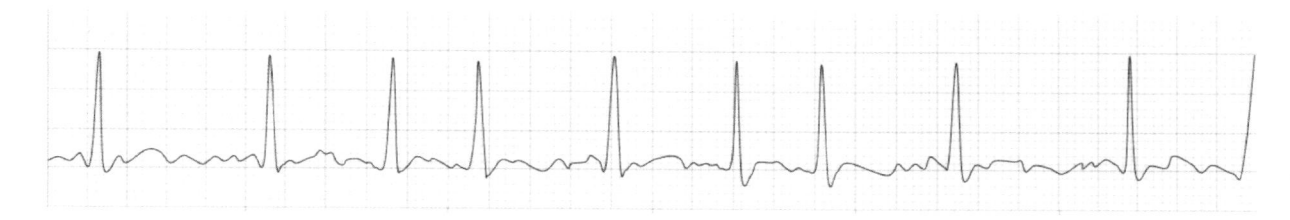

   a. The patient is in ROSC check responsiveness
   b. Perform synchronized cardioversion
   c. Resume CPR
   d. Perform defibrillation

48. Pauses in compressions should take no more than how long?
   a. 5 seconds
   b. 7 seconds
   c. 10 seconds
   d. 15 seconds

49. How long should a pulse and breathing check take?
   a. 1-2 seconds
   b. 3-6 seconds
   c. 5 seconds
   d. 5-10 seconds

50. What is the correct chest compression rate?
   a. 80/minute
   b. 100/minute
   c. 120/minute
   d. 100-120/minute

The Systematic Approach
(pp. 15-24 ACLS Provider Manual)

> • First check for a pulse and breathing if a patient appears unresponsive.

The systematic approach directs patient assessment. Form an initial impression from visual cues i.e., level of consciousness, awareness, and level of distress. Unconscious/unresponsive patients require a Basic Life Support (BLS) assessment while conscious patients require a primary and secondary assessment.

BLS Assessment (p. 18 ACLS Provider Manual)

Check scene safety and responsiveness, shout for help to request an AED and activation of the emergency response system and assess for a pulse and breathing **(between 5 and 10 seconds)**. Consider reversible causes (Hs & Ts) as they may precipitate cardiac arrest.

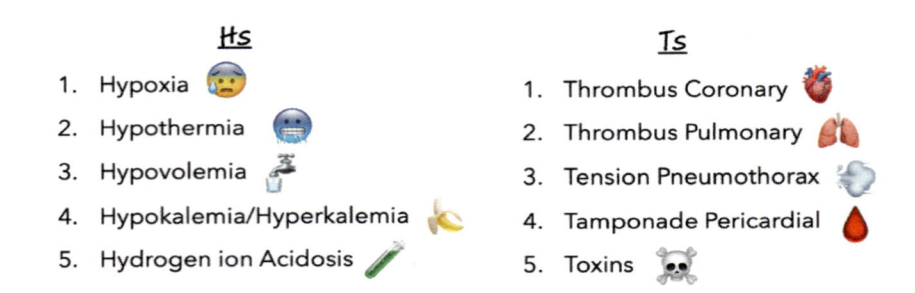

Hs	Ts
1. Hypoxia	1. Thrombus Coronary
2. Hypothermia	2. Thrombus Pulmonary
3. Hypovolemia	3. Tension Pneumothorax
4. Hypokalemia/Hyperkalemia	4. Tamponade Pericardial
5. Hydrogen ion Acidosis	5. Toxins

Primary Assessment (p. 21 ACLS Provider Manual)

The primary assessment evaluates **A**irway, **B**reathing, **C**irculation, **D**isability, and **E**xposure status. Recognize when life threats exist. Continually assess these until patient transfer. Manage per scope of practice and established protocols.

Secondary Assessment (pp. 22-23 ACLS Provider Manual)

The secondary assessment is a detailed evaluation utilizing the mnemonic SAMPLE, and consideration of the Hs & Ts. SAMPLE evaluates signs and symptoms, allergies, medications, past medical history, last oral intake, and preceding events. Further evaluate reversible causes through appropriate diagnostic measures.

Rapid Assessment

An expedient assessment technique to select the appropriate algorithm-based treatment involves asking three questions. The questions are (1) is a pulse present, (2) is the pulse fast or slow, and (3) is the patient stable or unstable. Review the patient assessment & treatment algorithm, which will be added to and referenced throughout the text.

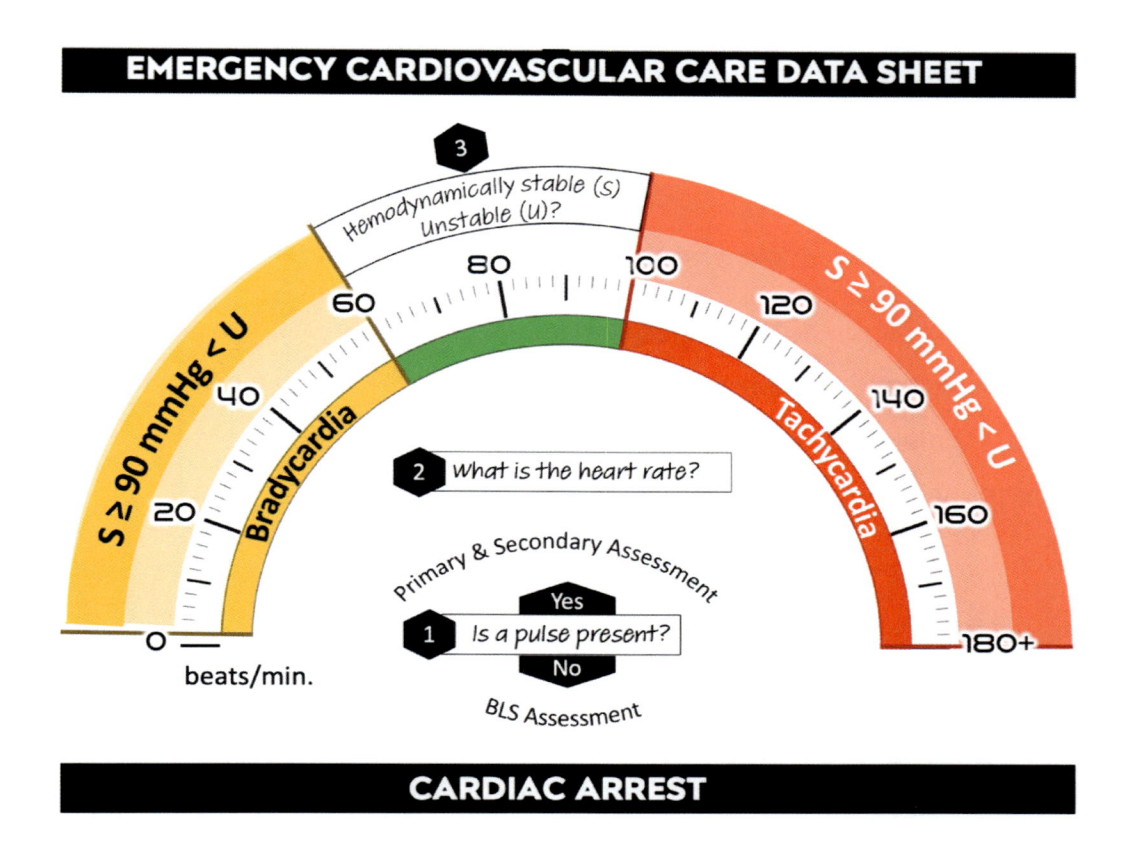

EMERGENCY CARDIOVASCULAR CARE DATA SHEET

3. Hemodynamically stable (S) / Unstable (U)?
- Bradycardia: S ≥ 90 mmHg < U
- Tachycardia: S ≥ 90 mmHg < U

2. What is the heart rate? (0–180+ beats/min.)

Primary & Secondary Assessment

1. Is a pulse present?
- Yes → Primary & Secondary Assessment
- No → BLS Assessment

CARDIAC ARREST

Systematic Approach

Basic Life Support
(pp. 17-20 ACLS Provider Manual)

> - Agonal gasps indicate cardiac arrest.
> - Ensure interruptions in chest compression do not exceed 10 seconds.
> - Perform chest compressions between 100-120 compressions per minute.
> - Immediately resume CPR beginning with chest compressions after defibrillation

BLS skills are foundational to advanced life support measures. Patients who are pulseless and apneic are in cardiac arrest and require high-quality cardiopulmonary resuscitation (CPR) to achieve a return of spontaneous circulation (ROSC). Certain criteria must be maintained to ensure high-quality BLS is being performed.

> - **Rate**: 100-120 compressions/minute.
> - **Depth**: 2 inches or 1/3 AP diameter of chest.
> - **Duration**: 2-minute cycles of chest compressions and breaths followed by a pulse and rhythm check.
> - **Ratio**: 30:2 compressions to breaths or continuous compressions and asynchronous respirations if advanced airway is present (ensure chest rise with breaths).

Chest Compression Effectiveness

Chest compression effectiveness is vital to maintaining high-quality CPR. Measure compression quality with feedback devices, a CPR coach, and exhaled carbon dioxide (PETCO2/ETCO2) readings. A PETCO2/ETCO2 reading of 10 mmHg indicates effective chest compressions, remember "PETCO2/ETCO2 of 8, CPR isn't great."

Chest compression effectiveness and time spent performing chest compressions i.e., chest compression fraction (CCF) is vital to obtain ROSC. Divide the amount of time spent performing chest compressions by the total resuscitation time to calculate CCF. High-performance teams maintain a minimum CCF above 80% by limiting pauses in compressions to 10 seconds or less and by **charging the defibrillator at the 1:45 minute mark**.

A 10% CCF increase equals an 11% increase for a return of spontaneous circulation. Adequate CCF supports coronary perfusion pressures (CPP). Perfused myocardial tissue responds to medications and electrical therapies.

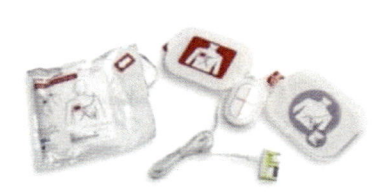

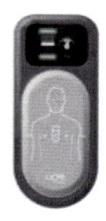

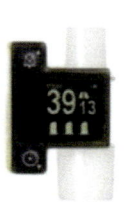

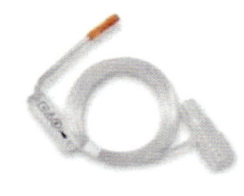

Pauses in compressions decrease CPP; the longer the pause the longer it takes to regain optimal CPP. Compare how CPP works to siphoning fluid from one container to another via a hand pump. The first few hand pump squeezes produce little to no fluid transfer.

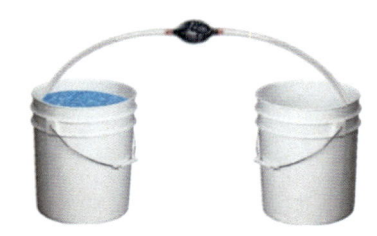

Consistent squeezes draw fluid into the pump until the volume can be ejected into the empty container. CPP steadily increases as chest compressions remain consistent. Coronary arteries fill during diastole while the rest of the body is perfused during systole.

CPP is the difference between Aortic Diastolic and Left Ventricular end-diastolic pressures (arterial line required). Target a mean arterial pressure (MAP) of > 65 mmHg to perfuse critical organs. Maximal CPP is the best factor for obtaining ROSC.

> ✅
> - What assessment is used for an unconscious patient?
> - What does SAMPLE stand for?
> - Reversible causes are also known as what?
> - Name 3 reversible causes.
> - Which questions quickly allow you to assess a patient's status?

BLS Skills Assessment Criteria

Students are expected to successfully perform Adult BLS. Passing requires completion of all the criteria found on the following page. Students can spend as much time as needed to practice the Adult BLS Assessment scenario.

Advanced Cardiovascular Life Support
Adult High-Quality BLS
Skills Testing Checklist

Student will be provided with a scenario either in a prehospital or hospital-based situation.

Assessment and Activation
- ☐ Checks responsiveness
- ☐ Shouts for help/Activates emergency response system/Sends for AED
- ☐ Checks breathing
- ☐ Checks pulse

Once student shouts for help, instructor says, "I am going to get the AED."

Compressions — Audio/Visual feedback device required for accuracy
- ☐ Hand placement on lower half of sternum
- ☐ Perform continuous compressions for 2 minutes (100-120/min)
- ☐ Compresses at least 2 inches (5 cm)
- ☐ Complete chest recoil. (Optional, check if using a feedback device that measures chest recoil)

Rescuer 2 says, "Here is the AED, I'll take over compressions and you use the AED."

AED (follows prompts of AED)
- ☐ Powers on AED
- ☐ Correctly attaches pads
- ☐ Clears for analysis
- ☐ Clears to safely deliver a shock
- ☐ Safely delivers a shock
- ☐ Shocks within 45 seconds of AED arrival

Resumes Compressions
- ☐ Ensures compressions are resumed immediately after shock delivery
  - Student directs instructor to resume compressions or
  - Second student resumes compressions

STOP TEST

Instructor Notes
- If the student does not complete all steps successfully (as indicated by at least 1 blank check box), the student must receive remediation.

Basic Life Support Performance

Cardiovascular System Review

The cardiovascular system circulates the entire blood supply (approximately 5-6 liters) within one minute. Blood is a complex connective tissue that delivers oxygen and nutrients to cells, transports waste from cellular metabolism, regulates temperature, facilitates immunological defenses, and serves as a buffer to regulate pH. A vascular network transports blood to every area of the body by way of the heart's pumping action.

The heart pumps blood by contracting its four chambers (right atria, right ventricle, left atria, left ventricle) rhythmically. Cardiomyocytes generate the electrical activity (automaticity) responsible for myocardial contraction. Automaticity follows an organized path through the heart to ensure effective contractions.

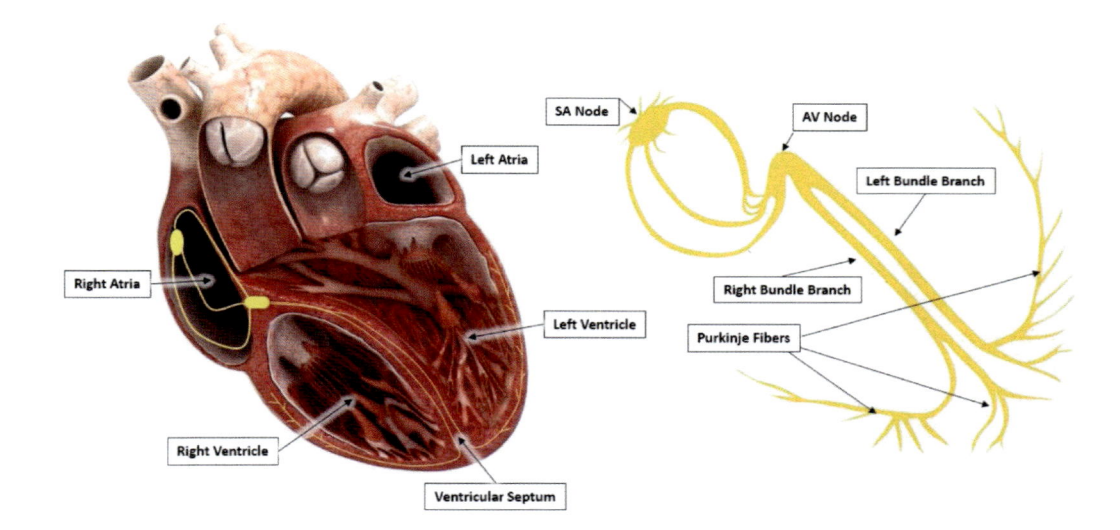

Cardiovascular Anatomy

The chief cardiomyocytes responsible for myocardial contraction are the sinoatrial (SA) node, atrioventricular (AV) node, bundle of HIS, and purkinje fibers (includes left and right bundle branches). Electrically charged ions shift across cellular membranes (cell wall) and cause myocardial contraction. Cellular membranes regulate the flow of ions between the intra/extracellular spaces until the membrane potential (electrical threshold) has been reached and depolarization occurs.

Intrinsic Cardiac Pacemaker Rates

Pacemaker	Rate beats/minute
SA node	60-100
Atrial foci	60-80
Junctional foci	40-60
Ventricular foci	20-40

Depolarization (a change in electrical charge) results in myocardial contraction. Relate cellular depolarization to firing a gun, where a trigger must travel a certain distance under the right amount of pressure before a handgun can fire. These depolarizations can be detected by way of an electrocardiogram (ECG).

> ✓
> - How long should pauses in compressions be kept to?
> - What is the required chest compression rate?
> - What is the adult compression depth?
> - PETCO2/ETCO2 of 10 mmHg indicates what?
> - Perform what action at the 1:45 minute mark to maximize CCF?

Cardiovascular Conduction System

ECG Interpretation

Successful navigation of the ACLS provider written examination and megacode high performance team activity requires ECG interpretation skills. There are numerous ECG considerations that will not be covered within this section pertaining to certain arrhythmias, axis deviation, and 12-lead ECG nuances. Lead II will serve as the primary point of reference for this chapter.

What is an ECG?

An ECG is a graphic representation of myocardial depolarizations over time. ECGs are produced by leads placed on a patient's body. ECGs are printed on graph paper illustrating time on the horizontal axis and electrical amplitude on the vertical axis.

ECG paper is composed of 1 mm x 1 mm squares denoting 0.1 mV and 0.04 seconds, which make up large 5 mm x 5 mm squares. ECG tracings capture either 6 seconds (30 large blocks) or 10 seconds (50 large blocks) of time. ACLS providers can acquire either a 3-lead or 12-lead ECG.

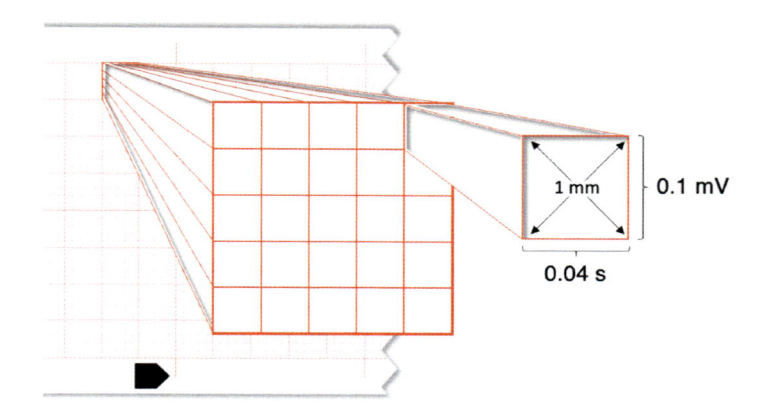

ECG tracings aid in identifying cardiovascular problems. Identification of normal ECG morphology helps distinguish an abnormal tracing. ACLS providers must recognize when an ECG is abnormal to render appropriate treatments.

What does a normal ECG look like?

ECG features include deflections either positive (upward) or negative (downward), segments, and intervals. Segments regard deviations in amplitude from the isoelectric line (baseline), whereas intervals measure time. Most people, when asked what an ECG looks like, would picture something like the adjacent image.

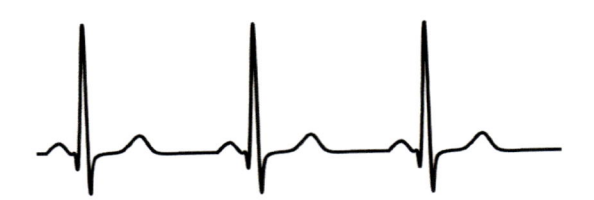

The above ECG rhythm, Normal Sinus Rhythm (NSR) viewed from lead II, is frequently depicted in television shows, advertisements, and logos, hence its familiarity to most people. Lead II has a favorable head-on view of the heart's electrical activity. To understand why the lead II perspective is favorable an understanding of how leads view the heart is essential.

How do leads create ECG tracings?

Lead II is one of 12 perspectives produced by a 12-lead ECG. Based on a lead's perspective the corresponding tracing may vary in appearance. Relate leads to seats in a baseball stadium. A spectator's perspective of how the ball travels may differ from another's who is seated in a different area.

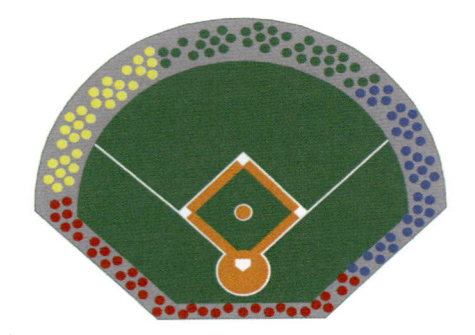

Spectators seated in the blue area, viewing a foul ball hit towards the red seating area along the third base line would see the ball moving away from them while those in the yellow area would generally see the ball traveling toward them until it came to rest in the red seating area. Conversely, a homerun heading toward the green seating area viewed by those seated in the green area would see the ball traveling directly at them just like lead II views electricity from the atria.

The baseball stadium analogy relates to how leads portray their view of electrical activity on ECG paper. A positive deflection in a lead means the flow of electricity is traveling toward that lead, whereas a negative deflection means the flow of electricity is traveling away from that lead. Examine the below image depicting lead placement with their vantage points aligning with the plus signs (+).

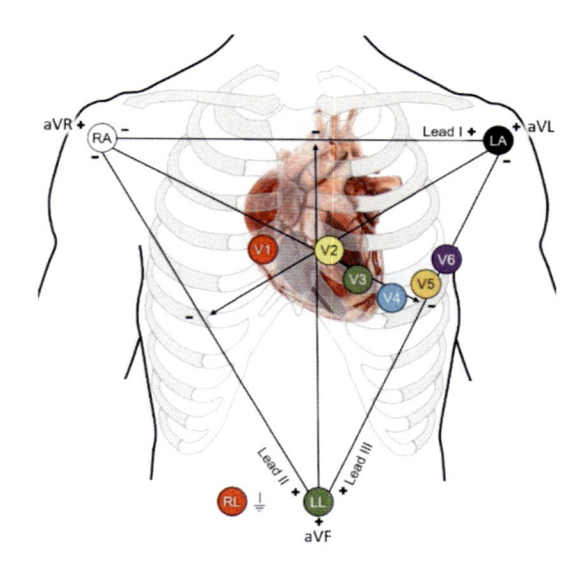

There are two types of leads, bipolar (having a positive and negative end) limb leads, and precordial leads. Limb leads view the heart in the frontal plane and include I, II, III, aVR, aVL, and aVF. Precordial leads view the heart in the transverse plane and include V1, V2, V3, V4, V5, and V6.

Linear movement is easy to assess, however the heart is a three-dimensional structure and electricity doesn't always flow linearly. Leads capture what they can see within the plane they are viewing, which is why multiple leads are used to view the entire heart. A lead's tracing depicts depolarizations as deflections starting with the SA node and terminating with the purkinje fibers.

This newfound understanding of how leads produce ECG tracings warrants further examination of NSR. Sinus means a rhythm originated from the sinoatrial node (SA node). NSR consists of the following elements: P-wave, PR segment, PR interval, QRS interval, ST segment, T wave, and QT interval.

Lead Placement

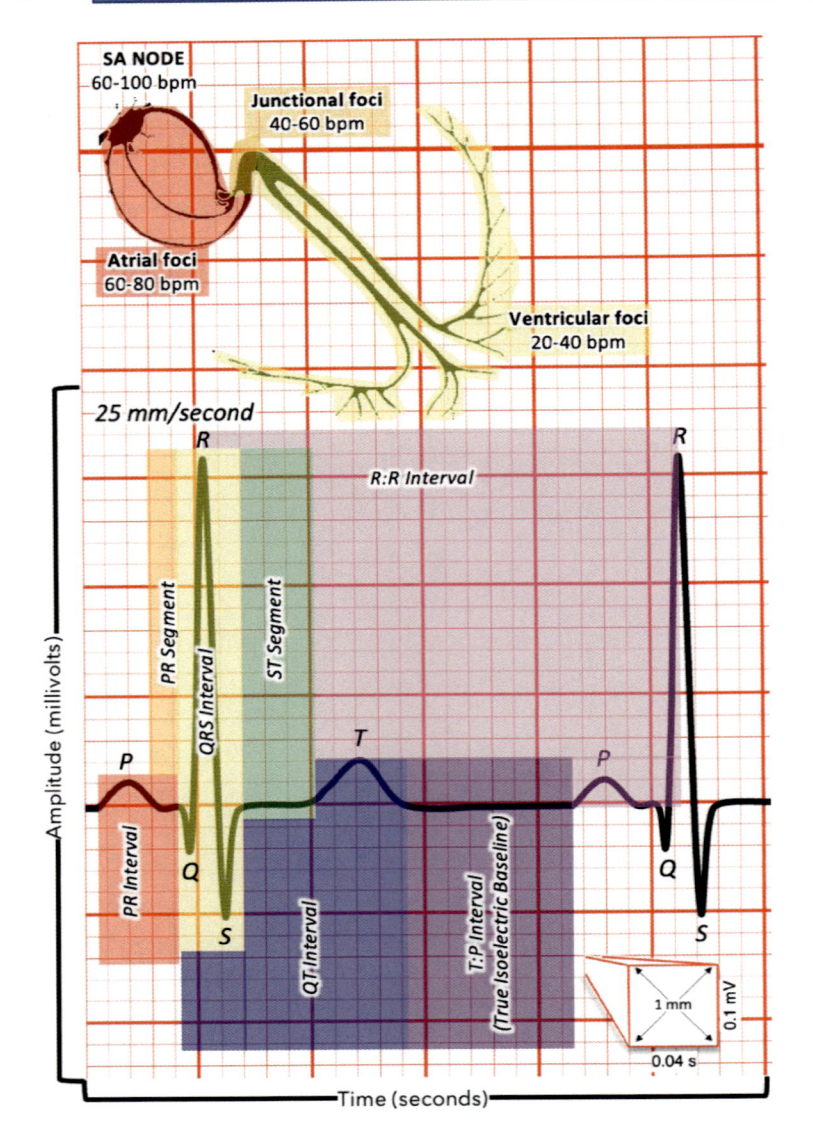

Normal Sinus Rhythm Parameters viewed from lead II	
Heart Rate:	60-100/min
P wave:	Atrial depolarization Amplitude: ≤ 2.5 mm Duration: < 0.12 s
PR Segment:	AV node depolarization, baseline for measuring ST elevation
PR Interval:	Time electricity takes to move through the atrium and the atrioventricular junction Duration: 0.12 s - 0.2 s
QRS interval:	Ventricular depolarization Duration: 0.06 s - 0.12 s **Q:** Ventricular septal depolarization **Amplitude:** ≤ 1/3 of R wave amplitude **R:** Apical ventricular depolarization **Amplitude:** ≤ 20 mm **S:** Basal ventricular depolarization
ST segment:	1 mm elevation in two contiguous leads other than V2, and V3 (2 mm).
T wave:	Ventricular repolarization **Amplitude:** 6 mm
QT interval:	QT ≤ 0.40 s @ 70 bpm; for every 10 bpm ▲ 70 subtract 0.02 s, and for every 10 bpm ▼ 70 add 0.02 sec

ECG Interpretation

Dysrhythmia (bad rhythm) and arrhythmia (no rhythm) are generally used interchangeably to describe an abnormal heart rate or rhythm. Analyze ECGs to distinguish dysrhythmias in a consistent manner to avoid misinterpretation with NSR serving as the point of reference. Examine the heart rate, regularity, PR interval, and QRS interval.

Determine Heart Rate

The normal adult heart rate is 60-100 beats per minute (bpm), less than 60 bpm is bradycardia, above 100 bpm is tachycardia, and above 150 bpm is supraventricular tachycardia (SVT). Two methods to calculate heart rate are the multiplication method, and the division method. A case can be made for each method's utility.

Multiplication Method

Count the number of R-waves on the strip and multiply that number by 10 for a 6 second strip or by 6 for a 10 second strip. The multiplication method is useful if there are relatively few R waves on the ECG tracing. When R waves are too numerous to count, use the division method.

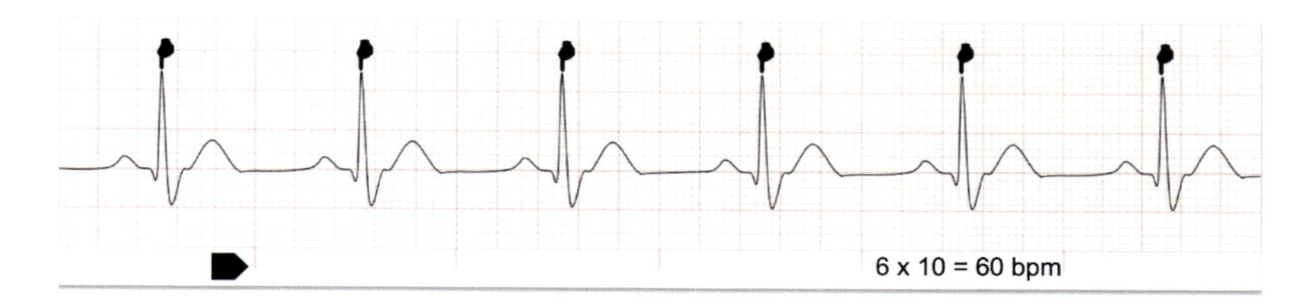

6 x 10 = 60 bpm

Division Method

A paper speed of 25 mm/second is 300 large blocks per minute (10 s. strip 50 x 6 or 6 s. strip 30 x 10). One R-wave for every large square (300/1) is 300 bpm and one every two large squares (300/2) is 150 bpm. When R-waves do not line up at large square intervals, dividing by a decimal where each little square equal 0.2.

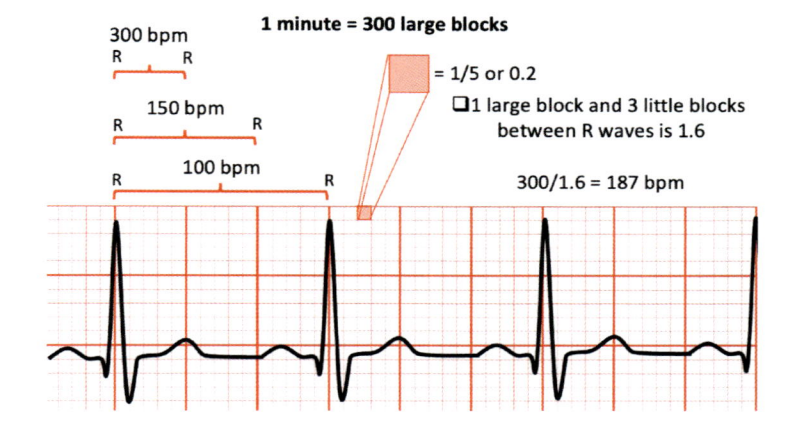

1 minute = 300 large blocks

300 bpm
R R

150 bpm
R R

100 bpm
R R

= 1/5 or 0.2

❑ 1 large block and 3 little blocks between R waves is 1.6

300/1.6 = 187 bpm

Regularity

Regular rhythms have even spacing between R waves (R:R interval), while irregular rhythms have variable R:R intervals. Waveforms can be described as regular, irregular, regularly irregular, or irregularly irregular. Regularly irregular waveforms have variable R:R intervals but follow a pattern (Second degree AV Block Type I), while irregularly irregular waveforms have variable R:R intervals and do not follow a pattern (atrial fibrillation, wandering atrial pacemaker, multifocal atrial tachycardia).

```
  1       1       1      .25  1   .5 .25  1
┌───┐   ┌───┐   ┌───┐   ┌┬┐  ┌─┐ ┌┬┬─┐
RegulaR  RegulaR  iRRegulaR  iRRegulaR
```

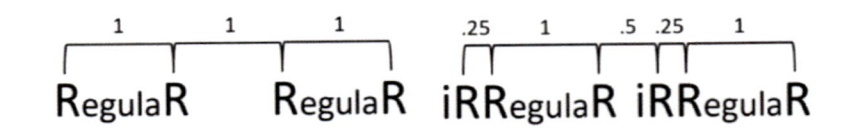

PR Interval

The PR interval represents the amount of time it takes an electrical impulse to travel through the atria and the atrioventricular junction. An elongated PR interval indicates that there is a delay in conduction and may indicate the presence of an atrioventricular (AV) block. Examine PR interval length and consistency to differentiate different arrhythmias.

A waveform with a PR interval greater than one large block (0.2 s.), absent other morphology, indicates the presence of a First-Degree heart block. A PR interval that gradually lengthens until a QRS complex drops is a Second-Degree AV Block Type I. A completely variable PR interval with a consistent P:P and R: R intervals with more P waves than QRS complexes is a Third-Degree AV Block.

QRS Interval

The QRS interval represents ventricular depolarization and should not exceed 3 small blocks (0.12 s.) in duration. A QRS interval greater than 3 small blocks is considered wide. If a stable patient presents with a wide QRS request immediate expert consultation.

> ✓
> - Where does a sinus rhythm originate?
> - One small block equals how many seconds?
> - One large block equals how many seconds?
> - What is the normal adult heart rate?

ECG Interpretation

Algorithms

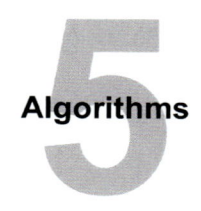

ACLS directs ECC through algorithm-based treatments. The algorithms a provider must know include Cardiac Arrest (VF/pVT & PEA/Asystole), Bradycardia, Tachycardia, Post Cardiac Arrest Care (ROSC), Acute Coronary Syndrome (ACS), and Stroke. Use of the emergency cardiovascular care data sheet introduced in chapter one will help determine the appropriate algorithm to use. Individual sections from the data sheet will be introduced with their respective algorithm. The portions of the data sheet will include the following icons:

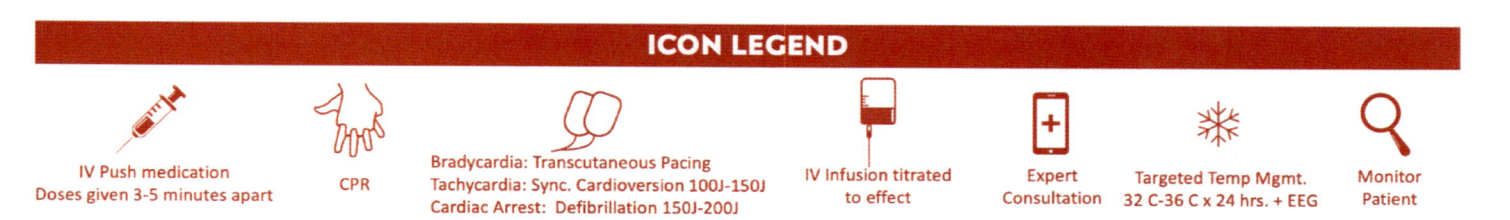

ICON LEGEND

- IV Push medication — Doses given 3-5 minutes apart
- CPR
- Bradycardia: Transcutaneous Pacing / Tachycardia: Sync. Cardioversion 100J-150J / Cardiac Arrest: Defibrillation 150J-200J
- IV Infusion titrated to effect
- Expert Consultation
- Targeted Temp Mgmt. 32 C-36 C x 24 hrs. + EEG
- Monitor Patient

Hemodynamic stability i.e., symptomatic (unstable) or asymptomatic (stable) directs the degree of care. Unstable patients may present with hypotension, an altered level of consciousness, signs of shock, chest pain/discomfort, or acute heart failure. Regardless of the algorithm used, always identify, and treat potential underlying causes (Hs & Ts).

> ⚠️ **Obtain the following for every patient**
> - 12-lead ECG
> - Vital Signs
> - IV Access
> - Oxygen on standby
> - Consideration of advanced airway management

Pharmacology

Administer injections every 3-5 minutes and infusions over 10-20 minutes titrated for effect. Cardiovascular drug interactions fall into one of three types: inotropic, chronotropic, or dromotropic, whereby a drug can have multiple effects.

- Inotropes affect cardiac contractile force.
- Chronotropes affect heart rate.

- Dromotropes affect electrical conduction velocity.

The following medication list is not comprehensive; however, it includes all the pertinent cardiovascular medications utilized during the high-performance team megacode activity. A 20 mL flush should follow intravenous push medications. Ensure that the IV line is stopped between the medication port and IV bag while administering the medication.

Adenosine (Adenocard) is used in the tachycardia algorithm because the heart rate is fast, and it needs to be slowed down and A<u>d</u>enosine has a "d" for down.
<u>Stable tachycardia:</u> 6 mg IV rapid push first dose, 12 mg IV rapid push second dose.

Amiodarone (Cordarone) is used in the cardiac arrest algorithm because if someone's heart stops you would probably say "Oh no!" which rhymes with Amio.
<u>Cardiac arrest:</u> 300 mg IV/IO first dose, 150 mg IV/IO second dose.

Atropine is used in the bradycardia algorithm because the heart rate is slow, and it needs to be plus'd up, and A<u>t</u>ropine has a T which looks like a plus sign.
<u>Bradycardia:</u> 1 mg IV/IO doses every 3-5 minutes up to a maximum of 3 mg.

Dopamine second line treatment for bradycardia and hypotension, avoid use with sodium bicarbonate.
<u>Bradycardia:</u> 5-20 mcg/kg/min infusion titrated to effect.

Epinephrine used in both cardiac arrest and in unstable bradycardia
<u>Cardiac arrest:</u> 1 mg (10 mL of 0.1 mg/mL solution) every 3-5 minutes.
<u>Unstable bradycardia:</u> 2-10 mcg/min infusion titrated to effect.

Lidocaine suppresses automaticity and increases electrical stimulation threshold.
<u>Cardiac arrest:</u> 1-1.5 mg/kg IV/IO first dose, then 0.5-0.75 mg/kg IV/IO at 5–10-minute intervals until a maximum dose of 3 mg/kg.

Magnesium Sulfate not routinely used during cardiac arrest unless Torsades de Pointes is suspected. Ensure QT interval is prolonged, normal QT interval with polymorphic tachycardia suggests need for alternative treatment.
<u>Cardiac arrest:</u> (polymorphic VT-Torsades de Pointes): 1-2 g IV/IO diluted in 10 mL D5W as bolus over 20 minutes.

Medication Type	Mechanism of Action	Medications
Inotropic	Positive (+) effects increase contractile force Negative (-) effects decrease contractile force	• Adenosine (-) • Dopamine (+) • Epinephrine (+) • Lidocaine (-) • Magnesium Sulfate (-)
Chronotropic	Positive (+) effects increase heart rate Negative (-) effects decrease heart rate	• Adenosine (-) • Amiodarone (-) • Atropine (+) • Dopamine (+) • Epinephrine (+) • Lidocaine (-) • Magnesium Sulfate (-)
Dromotropic	Positive (+) effects increase conduction velocity Negative (-) effects decrease conduction velocity	• Adenosine (-) • Amiodarone (-) • Atropine (+) • Dopamine (+) • Lidocaine (-) • Magnesium Sulfate (-)

✓
- Which 'A' named medications belong to the following algorithms:
    - Cardiac Arrest
    - Tachycardia
    - Bradycardia
- What is the first and second dose of amiodarone?
- Epinephrine administration is spaced out by how many minutes?

ACLS Pharmacology

Cardiac Arrest (pp. 115-149 ACLS Provider Manual)

> - Prompt defibrillation takes priority if cardiac arrest is assessed followed immediately by chest compressions.
> - Give epinephrine 1 mg following 2 defibrillation attempts.
> - Give Amiodarone 300 mg after epinephrine administration, generally after the third defibrillation attempt.
> - Increase chest compression fraction by charging your defibrillator 15 seconds prior to completing a rhythm check.
> - Any non-shockable pulseless ECG rhythm requires epinephrine 1 mg every 3-5 minutes.
> - A patient in pulsatile ventricular tachycardia who becomes pulseless requires immediate defibrillation.
> - The first dose of amiodarone during cardiac arrest is 300 mg.
> - Immediately defibrillate patients in ventricular fibrillation.

The cardiac arrest algorithm is considered the most important algorithm to know because it is the most utilized algorithm. The cardiac arrest algorithm has two pathways, the Ventricular Fibrillation/Pulseless Ventricular Tachycardia (VF/pVT) pathway and the Asystole/Pulseless Electrical Activity (PEA) pathway. Cardiac arrest has one of two outcomes, death, or Return of Spontaneous Circulation (ROSC).

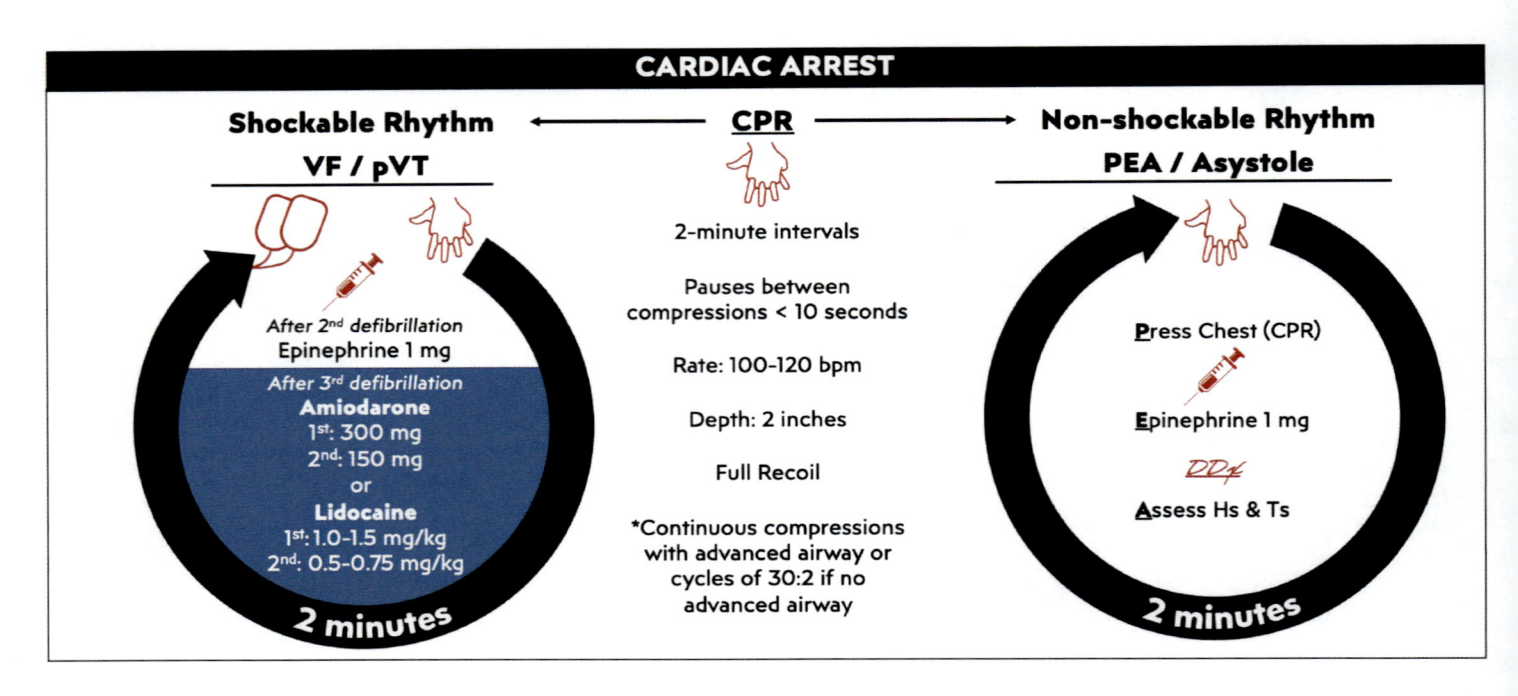

CARDIAC ARREST

Shockable Rhythm ← CPR → **Non-shockable Rhythm**
VF / pVT | | **PEA / Asystole**

Shockable Rhythm (VF / pVT) — 2 minutes:
- After 2nd defibrillation: Epinephrine 1 mg
- After 3rd defibrillation: Amiodarone
  - 1st: 300 mg
  - 2nd: 150 mg
  - or Lidocaine
    - 1st: 1.0-1.5 mg/kg
    - 2nd: 0.5-0.75 mg/kg

CPR:
- 2-minute intervals
- Pauses between compressions < 10 seconds
- Rate: 100-120 bpm
- Depth: 2 inches
- Full Recoil
- *Continuous compressions with advanced airway or cycles of 30:2 if no advanced airway

Non-shockable Rhythm (PEA / Asystole) — 2 minutes:
- **P**ress Chest (CPR)
- **E**pinephrine 1 mg
- ~~DDx~~
- **A**ssess Hs & Ts

A patient who achieves ROSC, whether the heart rate be fast or slow, is treated under the Post Cardiac Arrest Care algorithm. Avoid the urge to treat a slow or fast rhythm with the bradycardia or tachycardia algorithms respectively. Maintain the following criteria for individuals in cardiac arrest regardless of the pathway they are in.

- High-quality CPR in 2-minute intervals followed by a pulse/rhythm check.
- Limit compression interruption to less than 10 seconds.
- Resume compressions immediately after defibrillation attempts/pulse and rhythm checks.

VF/pVT Pathway

The VF/pVT pathway, also known as the shockable pathway, utilizes defibrillation (shocks) to eliminate abnormal cardiac rhythms. Defibrillation is administered at 360 Joules (J) for monophasic defibrillators or 150-200 J for biphasic defibrillators. Remember the VF/pVT pathway with the pneumonic "Shock, Shock, Everybody, Shock, ALabama."

Medications within this algorithm can be administered as soon as IV access has been achieved. Epinephrine has no max dose, while amiodarone and lidocaine can only be given twice and not together. Lidocaine blocks cardiac sodium channels shortening the action potential and amiodarone is a potassium channel-blocker that decreases cardiomyocyte excitability.

There are three specific waveforms significant to this pathway, monomorphic ventricular tachycardia, polymorphic ventricular tachycardia (including Torsades de Pointes), and ventricular fibrillation. When distinguishing between monomorphic and polymorphic tachycardia you do not have to overly scrutinize the ECG as it will be apparent.

Monomorphic VT

Monomorphic VT is very distinct, described as the grim reaper or tombstones. Monomorphic waveforms keep a consistent shape where the only visible peak is the R Wave. This is considered a wide complex tachycardia.

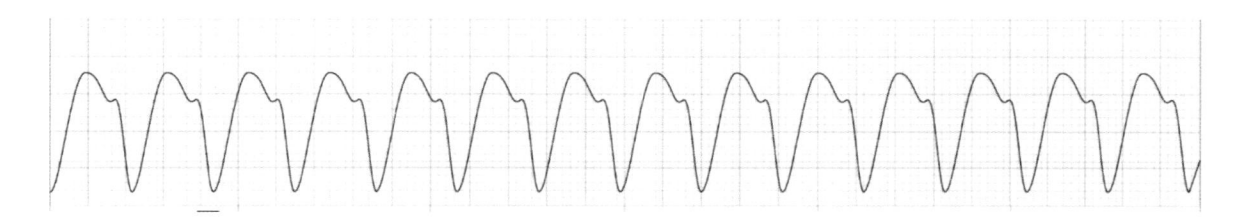

Polymorphic VT

Polymorphic ventricular tachycardia, by the virtue of the name poly- (many) morphic- (shape), has many different shapes. This waveform can have both low and high amplitudes and variable width QRS complexes.

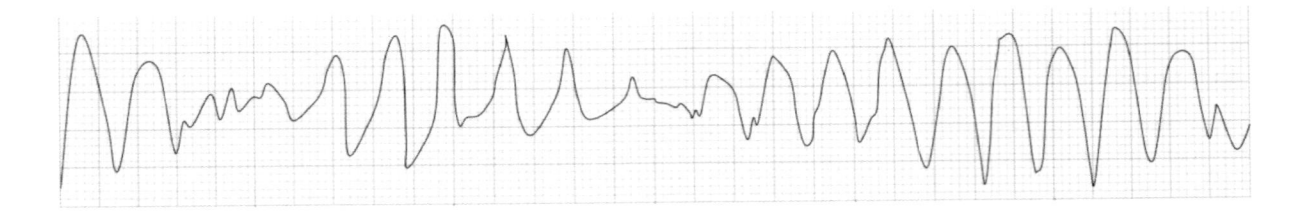

Torsades de Pointes

Torsades de Pointes is French for 'twisting of the points. It is described as having a spindle-like appearance. Torsades is a type of polymorphic VT that is treated with defibrillation and magnesium sulfate.

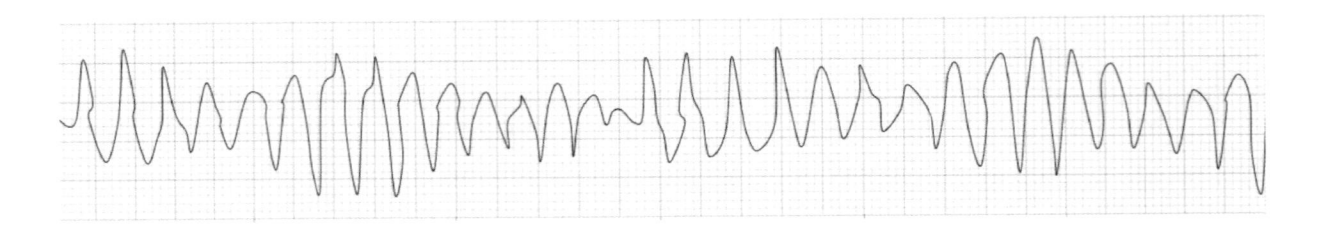

Ventricular Fibrillation

VF is a low amplitude, continuous squiggle. VF is a chaotic and disorganized rhythm without a discernable pattern. VF is always pulseless, remember "DEFIB the Vfib."

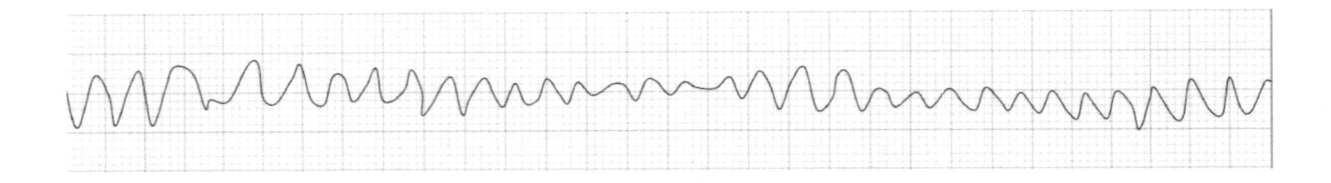

Asystole/Pulseless Electrical Activity Pathway

Any PULSELESS waveform, except VF/pVT, is considered pulseless electrical activity (PEA) and is treated under the cardiac arrest algorithm. The Pulseless Electrical Activity (PEA)/Asystole algorithm is for patients in cardiac arrest whose ECG rhythm is non-shockable. Interventions are limited to CPR, 1mg epinephrine injections, and consideration of reversible causes. Asystole, also referred to

> - Which medication follows the second defibrillation attempt?
> - What action immediately follows defibrillation/pulse and rhythm check?
> - What action increases CCF?
> - A patient in VF requires what treatment?
> - Which medication is an alternative to amiodarone?

as flat line, means that there is zero electrical activity. Remember we treat PEA with PEA (Press chest, Epinephrine, Assess Hs & Ts). Charge the defibrillator in the event a shockable rhythm appears during the rhythm check.

Cardiac Arrest Rhythms
Cardiac Arrest Algorithm

Bradycardia (pp. 66-74 ACLS Provider Manual)

- Identify a second-degree type I atrioventricular block.
- Identify a second-degree type II atrioventricular block.
- Identify a third-degree atrioventricular block.

Bradycardia is a heart rate below 60 beats per minute and considered clinically treatable below 50 beats per minute. Monitor hemodynamically stable patients for decompensation and treat hemodynamically unstable patients with the most appropriate therapy given the urgency of the situation. If intravenous access can be accomplished in a reasonable amount of time, administer Atropine (1 mg q 3-5 mins. max dose of 3 mg) and/or pharmaceutical pacing (infuse 2-10 mcg/min epinephrine or 5-20 mcg/kg/min dopamine over 10-20 minutes), otherwise perform transcutaneous pacing (consider sedation).

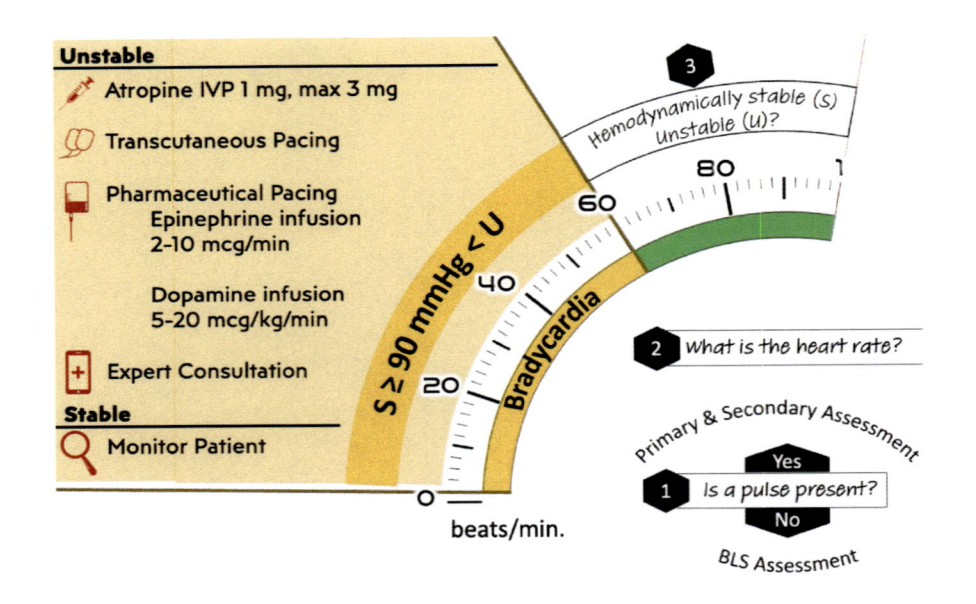

Pharmaceutical pacing has shown to be equally effective as transcutaneous pacing. The final step is to request expert consultation. You must be able to identify the following arrhythmias which are treated under the bradycardia algorithm.

- Sinus Bradycardia – resembles NSR but the heart rate is below 60 bpm
- Atrioventricular (Heart) Blocks
    - First Degree
    - Second Degree Type I
    - Second Degree Type II
    - Third Degree

Sinus Bradycardia

A waveform free from ectopy (electrical impulse originating outside of the SA-node) and below 60 bpm is considered sinus bradycardia. Clinically treatable bradycardia is generally below 50 bpm.

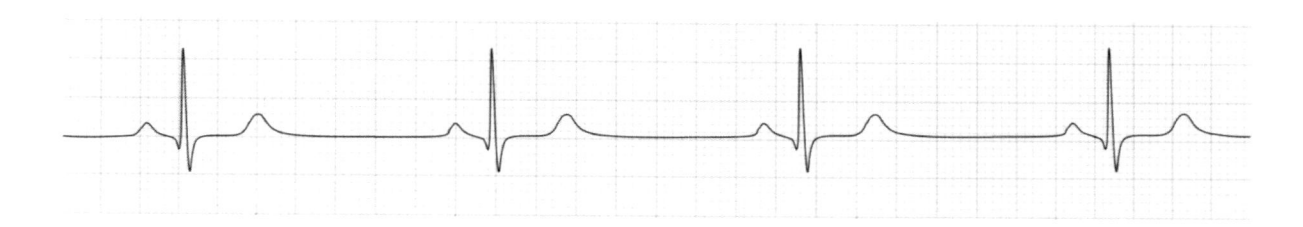

Heart Blocks

A heart block is a miscommunication of electrical activity between the atria and ventricles. There are different degrees of heart blocks i.e., first degree, second degree, and third degree. Second-degree heart blocks are further divided into type-1 or type-2. Relate heart blocks to dating relationships, imagine you are the P-wave, and your significant other is the QRS-complex.

First Degree Heart Block – "The Dependable Relationship"

Dependable relationships are reliable, communication is good, and where one goes so does the other. Sometimes even healthy couples need a little space, this can be seen with first degree heart blocks. A first-degree block is normal in every aspect except it has an increased PR-interval (≥ than 1 large block, 0.2 seconds).

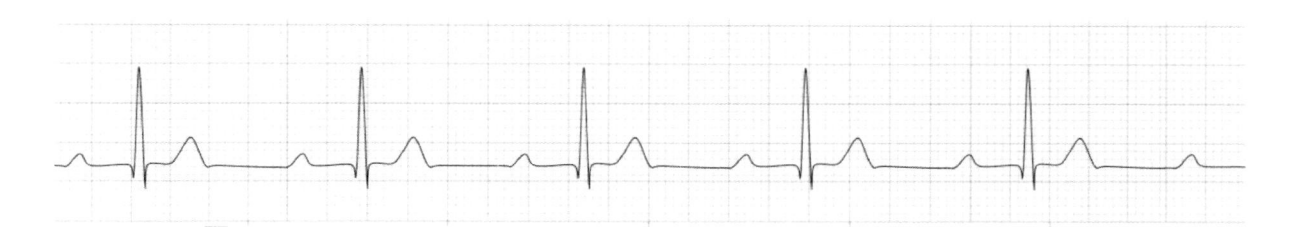

Second Degree Type-1 Heart Block – "The *Blind Date*"

Blind dates start with high hopes; however, blind dates can end poorly, and a second date is not in the cards. Second-Degree Type-1 Heart Blocks are like a bad blind date. The date starts well (PR-interval < 1 large box). The date takes an unexpected turn when you think you saw your date pick their nose, so you pull back a little (PR-interval increases). As the date progresses your date does it again, so you pull back even more. Finally, a second date doesn't happen (QRS falls off). The PR-interval gradually increases until the QRS falls off during second-degree type I heart blocks.

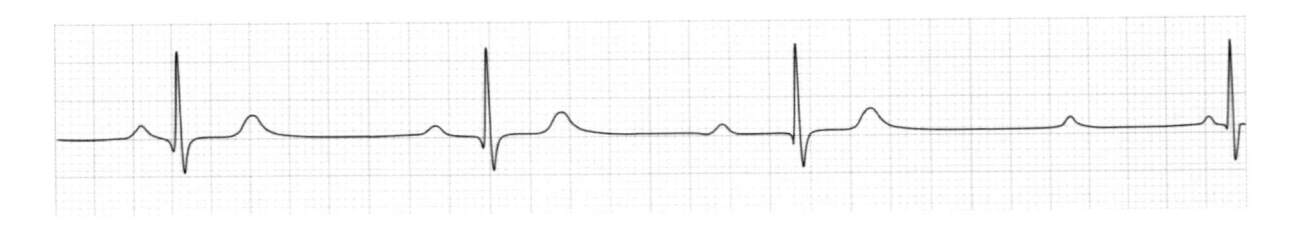

Second Degree Type-2 Heart Block – "The on Again-Off Again Relationship"

Some couples date and break-up and date again at different periods. Determining when a break-up happens is unpredictable. Things work normally while dating but can abruptly end without warning. Second-degree Type II heart blocks present normally but the QRS-complex unpredictably and randomly falls off.

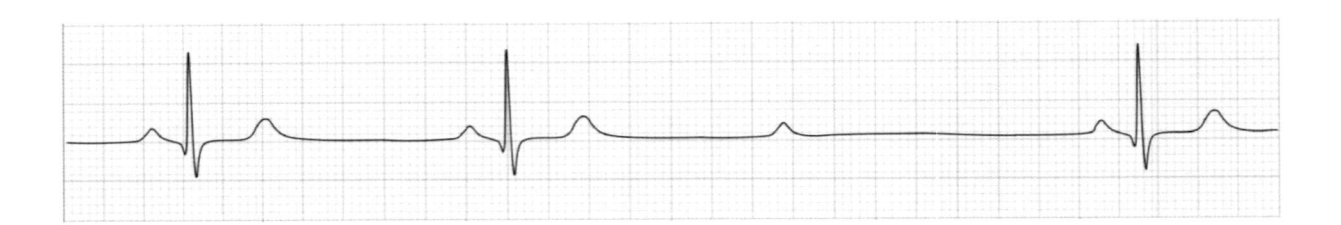

Third Degree Heart Block – "The Dysfunctional Relationship"

Individuals in dysfunctional relationships never seem to be on the same page. Agreement on a topic is probably sheer happenstance. Both parties do their own thing, miscommunication defines the relationship. Third degree heart blocks present this way. The P-wave and the QRS complex are out of sync. The one reliable thing about a third-degree heart block is that the P:P and R–R interval stays the same length, but the atria and ventricles are out of sync.

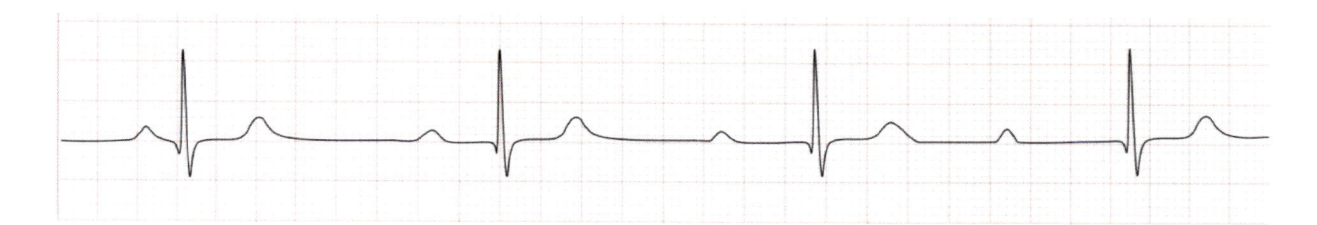

> ✓
> - What heart rate indicates bradycardia?
> - Which AV block has a consistent PR-interval > 0.2 seconds?
> - Which AV block has a PR-interval that increases until the QRS complex falls off?
> - What AV block looks normal except random QRS complexes drop-off?
> - Which AV block has consistent P:P and R:R intervals but has no relation between the P-waves and QRS complexes?

Bradycardia Rhythms
Bradycardia Algorithm

Tachycardia (pp. 75-89 ACLS Provider Manual)

- Identify monomorphic ventricular tachycardia (VT)
- Treat unstable pulsatile VT with synchronized cardioversion 100J-150J.
- Narrow-complex tachycardia refractory to adenosine requires a subsequent 12 mg dose of adenosine.
- Treat patients with pulsatile VT under the adult tachycardia with a pulse algorithm.
- An ECG tracing paired with a patient history is described by the patient's hemodynamic status i.e., stable, or unstable and the name of the rhythm. For example, a hypotensive patient in sinus tachycardia is defined as unstable sinus tachycardia.

Tachyarrhythmias exceed 100 beats per minute. Hemodynamically unstable patients require synchronized cardioversion between 100J-150J. Determine QRS width for stable patients, where a wide QRS is ≥ 0.12 seconds and requires expert consultation, if narrow < 0.12 seconds, perform vagal maneuvers, administer Adenosine (1st dose 6 mg, 2nd dose 12 mg), consider beta blockers, and request expert consultation.

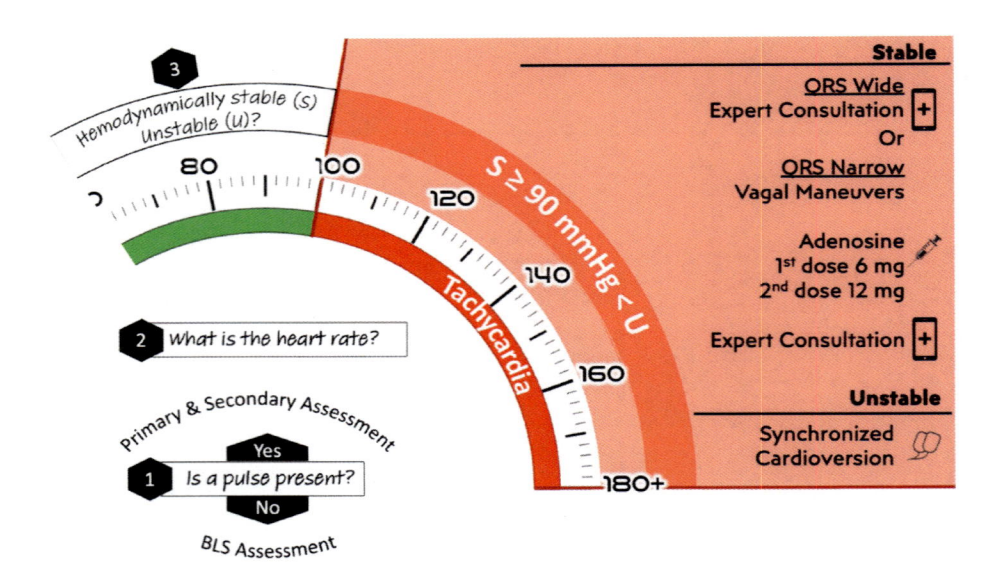

Stable
- QRS Wide — Expert Consultation
- Or
- QRS Narrow — Vagal Maneuvers
- Adenosine 1st dose 6 mg, 2nd dose 12 mg
- Expert Consultation

Unstable
- Synchronized Cardioversion

3. Hemodynamically stable (S) / Unstable (U)? S ≥ 90 mmHg < U Tachycardia
2. What is the heart rate? — Primary & Secondary Assessment
1. Is a pulse present? Yes / No — BLS Assessment

Remember from the cardiac arrest section that ventricular tachycardias can be pulseless as well as pulsatile. You must be able to identify the following arrhythmias which are treated under the tachycardia algorithm.

- Sinus Tachycardia
- Atrial Flutter
- Atrial Fibrillation
- SVT
- Ventricular Tachycardia (VT)
- Ventricular Fibrillation (VF)

Sinus Tachycardia

Sinus Tachycardia resembles NSR only faster. Rates between 100 and 150 bpm without ectopy are sinus tachycardia.

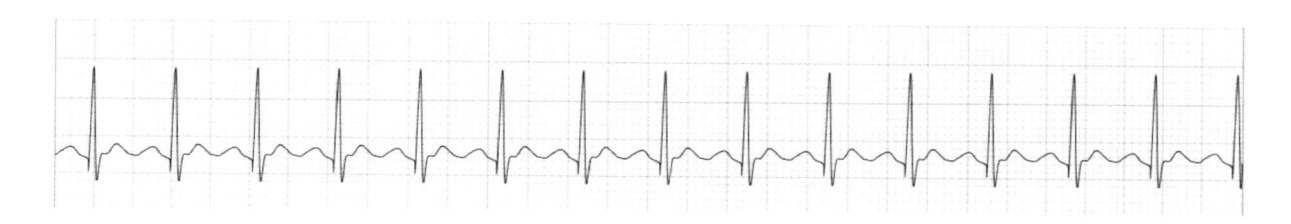

Atrial Flutter

Atrial flutter has a very pronounced saw tooth appearance with QRS complexes normally spaced throughout. The P Waves and T Waves are almost indistinguishable. The P-waves and T-waves almost resemble ventricular tachycardia with QRS-complexes evenly spaced throughout.

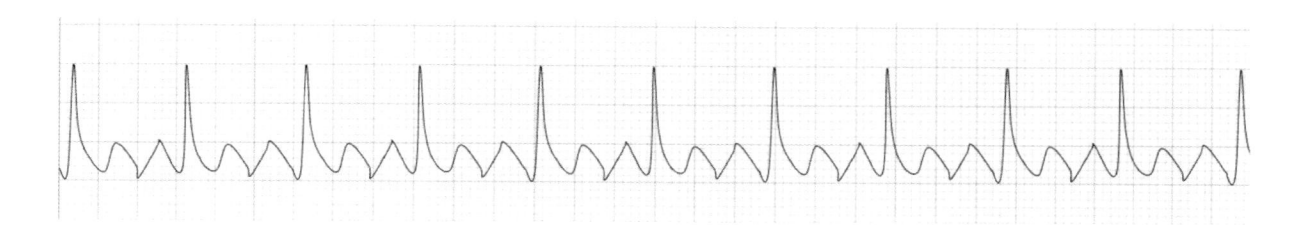

Atrial Fibrillation

Atrial fibrillation resembles a continuous squiggle with QRS complexes spaced regularly throughout. There are no distinguishable waves other than that of the R Wave in atrial fibrillation. This waveform resembles ventricular fibrillation with QRS-complexes evenly spaced throughout.

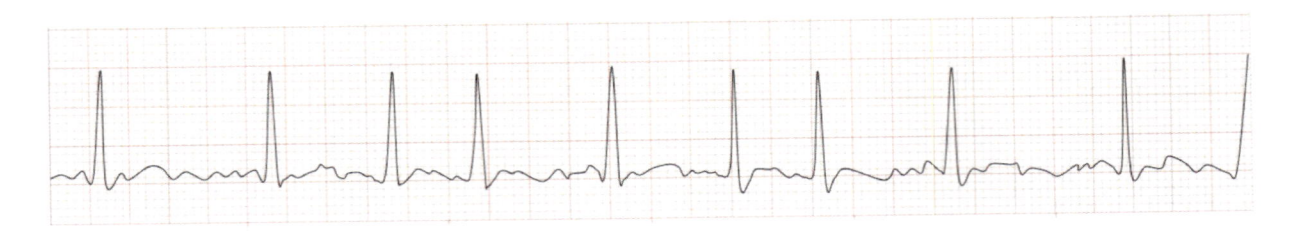

Supraventricular Tachycardia

SVT is a dysrhythmia where the heart rate is greater than 150 beats per minute. You may or may not be able to distinguish the presence of a P-wave. Normally this rhythm appears to be a string of QRS-complexes and T-waves. This is considered a narrow complex waveform.

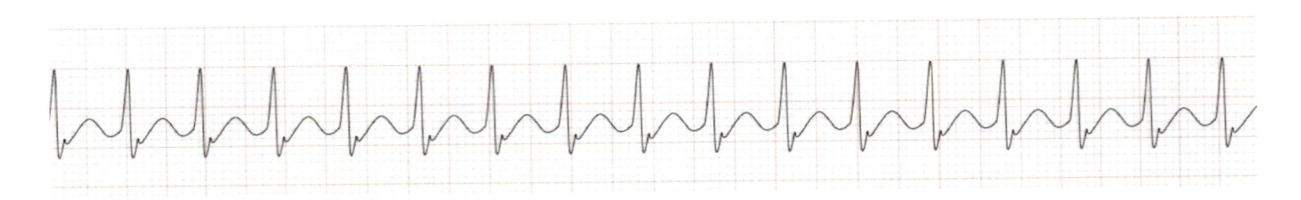

Ventricular Tachycardia

VT presents as a series of either monomorphic (one-shape) or polymorphic (many-shapes) wide QRS complex waveforms. Polymorphic VT will exhibit changes in amplitude and duration from one R Wave to the next, whereas monomorphic VT does not. Torsades de Pointes is a type of polymorphic VT that has a crescendo-like appearance that starts small, gradually increasing in size until it starts decreasing again; this is not the case in all instances of polymorphic VT.

- Tachyarrhythmias are over how many beats per minute?
- SVT exceeds what heart rate?
- What is a uniformly shaped VT called?

Tachycardia Rhythm
Tachycardia Algorithm

Post-Cardiac Arrest Care (pp. 150-159 ACLS Provider Manual)

> - Initiate and maintain targeted temperature management (TTM) for 24 hours for patients who achieve ROSC if unconscious/unable to follow commands.
> - Target a systolic blood pressure of 90 mmHg in during post cardiac arrest care for hypotensive patients.
> - Keep adult TTM between 32 and 36 degrees Celsius.

ROSC is achieved when a pulse returns in the absence of chest compressions, expect a concurrent rhythm change and a dramatic increase in PETCO2. Post cardiac arrest care focuses on monitoring the patient's status and investigating the cause of the cardiac arrest. Monitor level of consciousness, if unresponsive, initiate targeted temperature management 32° C – 36° C for 24 hours, perform advanced airway management, and request EEG monitoring. Monitor and maintain vital signs parameters per the below image. Lastly, investigate the cause of the patient's current state with diagnostic measures depicted in the image below.

POST CARDIAC ARREST CARE

MONITOR
Level of Consciousness: Conscious   Altered

Vital Signs
HR: 60-100
SBP: ≥ 90 mmHg
RR: 12-20, at least 10/minute
SPO2: 92%-98%
ETCO2: 35-45 mmHg

PRN

INVESTIGATE
12-Lead ECG
Radiology
CT/MRI/US/ECHO/Chest x-ray
Laboratory
ABG/Troponin/Cardiac Panel/ BUN

Acute Coronary Syndrome (ACS) (pp. 27-43 ACLS Provider Manual)

> - A 12-lead ECG takes priority for patients complaining of chest pain/discomfort.
> - Previous coronary artery stent placement indicates a prior acute coronary syndrome (ACS), which may be the cause of future chest pain/cardiac arrest.
> - Administer aspirin between 162 mg-325 mg to treat ACS.
> - Take cardiac arrest patients to cardiac reperfusion-capable medical centers only.
> - STEMI patients require percutaneous coronary intervention (PCI) within 90 minutes from their first medical contact.

ACS patients have a blockage of one or more coronary arteries. Rapid recognition of symptoms and activation of the emergency response system is vital. Chest pain is the primary symptom of ACS and indicates the need for a 12-lead ECG. ST segment elevation myocardial infarction (STEMI) on a 12-lead ECG confirms ACS. Give between 162 mg-325 mg aspirin.

The EMS transport team must notify the receiving facility prior to their arrival to prepare the catheter-lab, and only take ACS victims to facilities capable of providing Percutaneous Coronary Intervention (PCI). Initiate PCI within 90 minutes of first medical contact with the patient. Thrombolytic medications can be administered within 30 minutes after arrival at the medical facility.

Stroke (pp. 44-65, ACLS Provider Manual)

> - EMS expedite a suspected stroke patient's care by providing prearrival
> - Perform a non-contrast CT of the head less than 20 minutes after hospital arrival for suspected stroke patients.
> - Patients with a normal CT scan (ischemic stroke confirmation), whose symptoms started less than 3 hours ago, require fibrinolytic therapy ASAP.

Perform a physical and neurological examination. The NIH Stroke Scale (https://www.stroke.nih.gov/resources/scale.htm), Canadian Neurological Scale, and AHA/ASA Target Stroke: III all evaluate neurological status. A field expedient neurological evaluation is the F.A.S.T. acronym; **F**acial droop, **A**rm drift/weakness, **S**lurred speech, **T**ime to call 911/Time of onset.

The EMS transport team must notify the receiving neurovascular reperfusion capable facility of their ETA to activate the stroke team. Bypass the ED and go to the brain imaging suite (within 20 minutes). CT scans/MRIs distinguish between ischemic (87% of strokes) and hemorrhagic strokes. CT/MRI interpretation should occur within 30 minutes post arrival.

Ischemic strokes warrant IV thrombolytic use. Give IV thrombolytic (alteplase) within 3 hours from symptom onset (door-to-needle 60 mins). The rTPA window can be extended to four and a half hours for select patients. Patients' ineligible for thrombolytics require thrombectomy (door-to-device 90 minutes direct-arriving or 60 minutes transfer patients).

Airway Management
(pp. 100-113 ACLS Provider Manual)

> - Measure OPAs from the corner of the mouth to the angle of the mandible.
> - Confirm/monitor endotracheal tube placement via continuous waveform capnography.
> - Assess CPR quality via PETCO2 readings in intubated patients.
> - A PETCO2 reading of <10 mmHg indicates a need to improve chest compressions.
> - Treat hypoxia with oxygen.
> - Excessive ventilation decreases cardiac output.
> - Provide ventilation at one breath every six seconds.

Provide airway management based on patient status and scope of practice. Agonal gasps are not normal breathing and indicate cardiac arrest (perform chest compressions immediately). Maintain airway patency (openness) with a least to most invasive approach.

Place an unconscious patient in the supine (on back) position and perform the head-tilt-chin-lift/jaw thrust maneuver if breathing difficulty exists. Difficulty breathing unalleviated by repositioning may require bag mask ventilations and subsequent placement of an airway device. Begin with a simple airway adjunct and move to more advanced means if necessary.

Airway Management Devices

Oropharyngeal airways (OPAs) are for unconscious patients **ONLY** and are measured from the corner of the mouth to the angle of the mandible. Nasopharyngeal airways (NPAs) may be used in both conscious and unconscious patients and are measured from the nostril to the earlobe. Advanced airway placement i.e., endotracheal intubation, supraglottic airway devices is only for higher level medical practitioners.

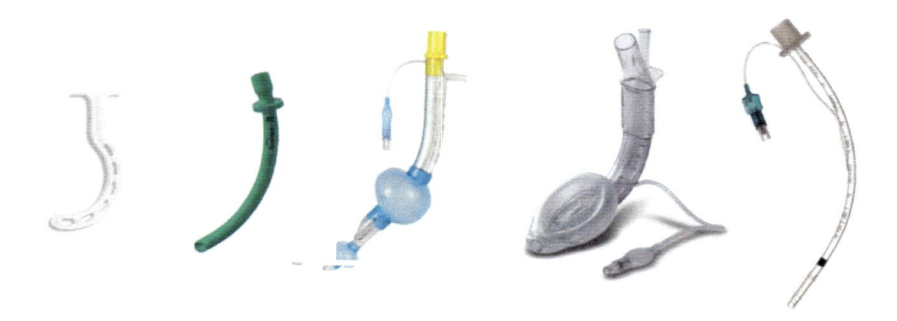

Capnometry and Continuous Waveform Capnography

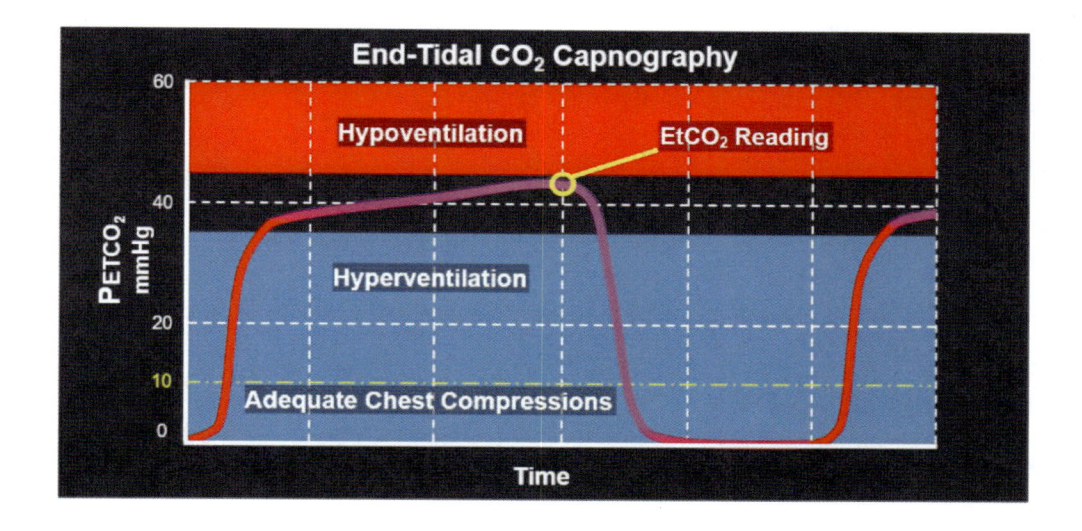

Capnometry was mentioned earlier regarding its use in measuring chest compression effectiveness, however the measurement of exhaled carbon dioxide can be used to ensure proper placement of endotracheal tubes. Continuous waveform capnography is the gold standard to ensure ETT placement not chest x-rays. Normal EtCO$_2$ is between 35-45 mmHg. A patient in cardiac arrest showing a dramatic increase in EtCO$_2$ may have regained a pulse. Figure 30 depicts normal continuous waveform capnography.

> ✓
> - Can an OPA be used to manage a conscious patient's airway?
> - How is an OPA measured?
> - What PETCO2 reading must be maintained to indicate effective compressions?
> - What is used to confirm endotracheal tube placement?
> - What is the normal PETCO2 range?

Airway Management Skills Assessment Criteria

During the Airway Management Assessment each student is expected to perform the following steps. Passing requires the student to not miss any of the below criteria. Students can spend as much time as needed to practice the Airway Management Assessment scenario.

Advanced Cardiovascular Life Support
Airway Management
Skills Testing Checklist

Critical Performance Steps	Check if done correctly
BLS Assessment and Intervention	
Checks for responsiveness Taps and shouts, "Are you OK?"	
Activates the emergency response system Shouts for nearby help/activates the emergency response system and gets the AED or Directs second rescuer to activate the emergency response system and get the AED	
Checks breathing Scans chest for movement (5-10 seconds)	
Checks pulse (5-10 seconds) **Breathing and pulse check can be done simultaneously** Notes that pulse is present and does not initiate chest compressions or attach AED	
Inserts oropharyngeal or nasopharyngeal airway	
Administers oxygen	
Performs effective bag-mask ventilation for 1 minute Gives proper ventilation rate (once every 6 seconds) Gives proper ventilation speed (over 1 second) Gives proper ventilation volume (about half a bag)	

STOP TEST

Instructor Notes

- If the student does not complete all steps successfully (as indicated by at least 1 blank check box), the student must receive remediation.

Airway Management

High-performance Teams
(pp. 91-163 ACLS Provider Manual)

> - High-performance team members assigned a role exceeding their scope of practice should ask for a new role.
> - Address team members immediately if they are about to make a mistake.
> - Medical Emergency Teams (METs)/Rapid Response Teams (RRTs) identify early clinical deterioration to improve patient outcomes.
> - If you are unsure of what was ordered, or if you feel the order was given incorrectly, by the team leader echo exactly as heard and ask if correct.
> - The CPR Coach ensures high-quality CPR is being conducted.
> - Responses to a given instruction should echo the instruction i.e., instruction: "draw up 300 mg amiodarone", response: "I will draw up 300 mg amiodarone."
> - Team leaders avoid resuscitation inefficiencies by clearly delegating tasks.

The final assessment an ACLS student must undergo is a high-performance team activity known as the Megacode. A high-performance team includes a Team Leader, Airway, IV/IO/meds, Compressor, Defib/Monitor, Recorder/Timekeeper, and CPR Coach. The CPR Coach is a new role first introduced in the 2020 ECC Guidelines and is responsible for ensuring high-quality CPR.

Resuscitation scenarios require teamwork and teamwork requires communication. Medical Emergency Teams and Rapid Response Teams exist to optimize patient outcomes by identifying and treating early deterioration. Team members must understand how to work and communicate effectively.

Closed Loop Communication: when a direction is given it should be echoed back to ensure a shared understanding is had and to identify inaccuracies.

Clear Roles and Responsibilities: each team member must understand their individual role on the team to ensure patient care is not delayed and that efforts are not being duplicated

Knowing Your Limitations: professional (scope of practice) and physical (disability related) boundaries exist for every team member. If you are asked to perform a Role that is outside of your professional or physical boundaries, ask for a new role.

Constructive Intervention: tactful and descriptive correction provided when a team member is about to incorrectly perform an action. For example, a team member notices that chest compressions are being performed at an inadequate depth, so he/she states, "chest compressions need to be 2 inches deep."

Knowledge Sharing: commonly misinterpreted for constructive intervention, is when someone becomes fixated on a course of action that may lead to an error, however team members provide open discussion to think of alternative treatment options.

> ✓
> - What is the purpose of METs and RRTs?
> - A team member unable to perform a task should do what?
> - Correcting a team member before they can make a mistake is known as what?
> - High-performance teams utilize what type of communication?
> - What is the CPR Coach's purpose?

The Megacode Overview

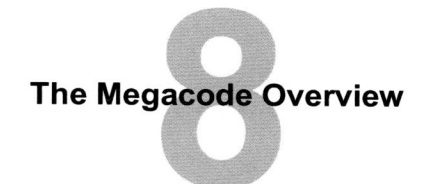

The megacode is a high-performance team activity where a team of individuals perform a resuscitation. The team must maintain a CCF above 80%, utilize effective communication techniques, and perform role-specific duties to pass the megacode test. Team members are permitted to use algorithm handouts during the megacode practice and testing scenarios.

Instructor Responsibilities

The instructor is a passive member during the activity to not influence the team's actions during practice and testing iterations. After the practice iterations the instructor will facilitate student discussion led debriefing. The instructor is responsible for performing the following:

- Pre-brief the team on megacode exercise expectations.
- Provide a realistic scenario.
- Provide feedback throughout the scenario as necessary without directly influencing what actions need to be taken by team members.
- Ensure debriefing is provided for both practice and testing scenarios.

Student Responsibilities

The instructor provided scenario will be one of 12 predetermined scenarios per the ACLS Instructor manual. The team is graded as a whole and thus passes or fails in kind. Individual performance as a team leader is not required to pass the megacode exercise. Students will be expected to perform all the responsibilities required of their assigned role. ACLS Instructors will evaluate the team's communication and acknowledgement of pertinent actions. Students should communicate effectively with their other team members; however, they should not lean on the competency of other students due to a personal lack of knowledge or understanding. Multiple practice scenarios will be presented where each student will rotate through the various team member roles. The following table outlines the performance points the team must meet.

Advanced Cardiovascular Life Support
Megacode Testing Checklist
Bradycardia/Tachycardia → Pulseless VT/VF → PEA → PCAC

Critical Performance Steps						Check if done correctly
Team Leader						
Assigns team member roles						
Ensures high-quality CPR at all times	Compression rate 100-120/min ☐	Compression Depth of >2 inches ☐	Chest compression fraction >80% ☐	Chest recoil ☐	Ventilation ☐	
Ensures that team members communicate well						
Bradycardia/Tachycardia Management						
Starts O2 if needed, places on monitor, obtains IV/IO access						
Places leads in proper position						
Distinguishes between a stable/unstable patient and properly identifies rhythm						
Provides correct 1st and 2nd line treatments						
Pulseless VT/VF Management						
Recognizes rhythm						
Clears before analysis and shock						
Immediately resumes CPR						
Appropriate cycles of drug-rhythm check/shock-CPR						
Administers appropriate drug(s) and doses						
PEA/Asystole Management						
Recognizes PEA						
Verbalizes potential reversible causes of PEA (H's and T's)						
Administers appropriate drug(s) and doses						
Immediately resumes CPR and rhythm checks						
Post-Cardiac Arrest Care						
Identifies ROSC						
Ensures BP and 12-lead ECG are performed and O2 saturation is monitored, verbalizes need for endotracheal intubation and waveform capnography, and orders laboratory tests						
Considers targeted temperature management						

STOP TEST

Instructor Notes

- If the student does not complete all steps successfully (as indicated by at least 1 blank check box), the student must receive remediation.

Vital Signs Differentiation

Hemodynamically unstable patients require treatment. The below parameters compare the difference between stable and unstable vital signs. Students must identify whether their patient is stable or unstable to select the appropriate treatment.

Vital Sign	Stable Values	Unstable Values
Heart Rate	60-100 bpm	< 60 or > 100 bpm
Blood Pressure	120/80 mmHg (SBP > 90 mmHg)	< 90 mmHg SBP
Respiratory Rate	12-20 breaths per minute	< 10 or > 24 breaths per minute
SPO2	92%-98%	< 92%
PETCO2/ETCO2	35-45 mmHg	< 35 mmHg alkalosis, > 45 mmHg acidosis
Pain	0 out of 10	Subjective

Example Megacode Scenario Transcript

Person/Event   **Statement**

Instructor: A 65-year-old male patient is brought to your emergency department by EMS transport. Your patient is clutching his chest in obvious discomfort, sweating profusely (diaphoretic), appears pale, weak, and is slightly confused about his whereabouts. How would you proceed with this patient?

This summary of symptoms is enough to direct the team to perform the initial therapies required (chapter 5 warning sign). The patient presents as unstable at first glance. Vital signs are not provided to the student until the student directs the appropriate treatments.

Team Leader: Let's acquire vital signs monitoring, a 12-lead ECG, initiate IV/IO access, and have oxygen on standby to treat hypoxia.

The instructor provides the appropriate vital signs and places a tachycardic rhythm on the monitor. The student must clear the patient for analysis and determine whether the patient is stable or unstable. An unstable tachycardic patient is what should be presented, and the team leader should direct for synchronized cardioversion between 100J-150J.

Team Leader: My patient has unstable tachycardia. Place the pads on the patient's chest and charge the monitor to 150J to perform synchronized cardioversion.

The team member on the monitor verbally confirms and carries out the order. The instructor verifies that the student set the monitor to sync and selects the directed energy dose. The instructor must ensure the student clears the patient prior to synchronized cardioversion delivery.

Defibrillator Role: Preparing for synchronized cardioversion at 150J. Charging.

[monitor charged]

Defibrillator Role: Everybody clear, shocking in 3, 2, 1.

[shock delivered]

Person/Event	Statement

The team leader watches the monitor for conversion to NSR. The instructor, immediately following synchronized cardioversion, places the patient into cardiac arrest by displaying ventricular fibrillation and informs the team that there has been a change in level of consciousness.

Instructor Your patient is now unconscious

Immediately recognizing that the patient is in cardiac arrest the team leader assigns team roles i.e., compressor, monitor/CPR Coach, airway, IV/IO access/meds, timekeeper/recorder, and initiates CPR. The team leader then directs the need for defibrillation, monophasic 360J or biphasic 150J-200J and initiates chest compressions.

Team Leader: Prepare to defibrillate the patient at 200J and begin CPR.

Compressor Role: Starting CPR.

The team member on the monitor verbally confirms and carries out the order, and prior to shock delivery, clears the patient and states "shocking in 3, 2, 1." Immediately after defibrillation the team leader directs for CPR to resume. The instructor must ensure that the team performs high-quality CPR.

Defibrillator Role: Preparing for defibrillation at 200J, charging.

[monitor charged]

Defibrillator Role: Everybody clear, shocking in 3, 2, 1.

[shock delivered]

Team Leader: Resume CPR and obtain advanced airway management.

Compressor Role: Resuming CPR.

Airway Role: Obtaining endotracheal intubation.

[airway obtained, does not interfere with compressions]

Airway Role: ETI achieved breathing one breath every six seconds.

Person/Event	Statement

[at 1:45]

Team Leader:	Charge the defibrillator to 200J and prepare 1 mg epinephrine but do not give it until directed.
Defibrillator Role:	Charging the monitor to 200J.

[monitor charges]

IV/IO/Meds Role:	Preparing 1 mg epinephrine

[2:00 minutes of CPR have elapsed]

The team leader or the timekeeper acknowledges when 2 minutes have elapsed and directs a pulse and rhythm check. Once two minutes have elapsed the instructor maintains pVT/VF on the monitor. The team leader recognizes VF and directs for defibrillation, resumption of CPR, and the administration of 1 mg epinephrine every 3-5 minutes.

Team Leader:	Check for a pulse.
Instructor:	No pulse present.
Team Leader:	Prepare to defibrillate.
Defibrillator Role:	Everybody clear, shocking in 3, 2, 1.

[shock delivered]

Team Leader:	Resume CPR, deliver 1 mg epinephrine.
Compressor Role:	Resuming CPR.
IV/IO/Meds Role:	Administering 1 mg epinephrine.

[IVP complete]

IV/IO/Meds Role:	1 mg epinephrine administered.

[at 1:45]

Team Leader:	Charge the defibrillator to 200J and prepare 300 mg amiodarone but do not give it until directed.
Defibrillator Role:	Charging to 200J.

Person/Event	Statement

[monitor charges]

IV/IO/Meds Role: Preparing 300 mg amiodarone.

[2:00 minutes of CPR have elapsed]

The team leader or the timekeeper acknowledges when 2 minutes have elapsed and directs a pulse and rhythm check. The instructor maintains pVT/VF on the monitor. The team leader recognizes VF and directs for defibrillation, resumption of CPR, and the administration of 300 mg amiodarone or 1-1.5 mg/kg lidocaine.

Team Leader: Check for a pulse.

Instructor: No pulse present.

Team Leader: Prepare to defibrillate.

Defibrillator Role: Everybody clear the patient, shocking in 3, 2, 1.

[shock delivered]

Team Leader: Resume CPR, deliver 300 mg amiodarone.

Compressor Role: Resuming CPR.

IV/IO/Meds Role: Administering 300 mg amiodarone.

[IVP complete]

IV/IO/Meds Role: 300 mg amiodarone administered.

[at 1:45]

Team Leader: Charge the defibrillator to 200J and prepare 1 mg epinephrine but do not give it until directed.

Defibrillator Role: Charging the monitor to 200J.

[monitor charges]

IV/IO/Meds Role: Preparing 1 mg epinephrine.

Person/Event	Statement

[2:00 minutes of CPR have elapsed]

After the Instructor verifies the students understanding of the pVT/VF pathway of cardiac arrest they will transition to the PEA/Asystole pathway. Once two minutes have elapsed the instructor places a non-shockable, pulseless rhythm on the monitor. The team leader recognizes the rhythm change, checks for a pulse and if absent directs dumping the charge due to PEA, resumes CPR, and the administration of 1 mg epinephrine.

Team Leader: Check for a pulse.

Instructor: No pulse present.

Team Leader: The patient is in PEA, resume CPR, dump the charge, and administer 1 mg epinephrine.

Compressor Role: Resuming CPR.

Defibrillator Role: Dumping the charge.

IV/IO/Meds Role: Administering 1 mg epinephrine.

[IVP complete]

IV/IO/Meds Role: 1 mg epinephrine administered.

The team recognizes that they need to consider potential reversible causes (Hs & Ts) hypothermia, hypoxia, hypovolemia, hypokalemia, hyperkalemia, hydrogen ion acidosis, thrombus coronary, thrombus pulmonary, tamponade cardiac, tension pneumothorax, toxins. Consideration of reversible causes can be indicated by any team member. The team should discuss the patient history and potential causative factors.

Team Leader: We need to consider potential reversible causes.

[Team discusses Hs & Ts and directs any appropriate diagnostics or treatments]

[at 1:45]

Team Leader: Charge the defibrillator to 200J.

Defibrillator Role: Charging the monitor to 200J.

[monitor charges]

[2:00 minutes of CPR have elapsed]

Person/Event	Statement

Once two minutes have elapsed the instructor places NSR on the monitor. The team leader recognizes the rhythm change and assesses for the presence of a pulse. The instructor indicates a pulse exists and the team leader verbalizes that ROSC has been achieved.

Team Leader: Check for a pulse.

Instructor: You have a pulse.

Team Leader: ROSC has been achieved, check the patient's level of consciousness.

Airway Role: The patient is unconscious.

Team Leader:
- Initiate targeted temperature management between 32-36 °C for 24 hours
- Obtain EEG monitoring.
- Monitor vital signs to achieve the following end states:
    - Heart rate: 60-100 bpm
    - Respiratory rate: no less than 10/minute
    - SpO2: 92-98%
    - Systolic blood pressure: no less than 90 mmHg
    - EtCO2: 35-45 mmHg

- Perform the following tests
    - 12-lead ECG
    - Chest x-ray
    - CT scan
    - Ultrasound
    - Echocardiogram
    - Troponin
    - ABG

This marks the conclusion of the megacode exercise. Throughout the event the instructor is reviewing for effective communication, and proper performance of all tasks. At the conclusion of the event the instructor will ask open-ended questions to spur conversation between the team members to identify things that went well and things that could have been improved. If the team maintained a CCF of at least 81%, and team members performed the responsibilities of their respective roles without using other team members as a crutch the team would be successful.

High-performance Team Activity

Posttest

1. How much aspirin would a telecommunicator direct a rescuer to administer for someone complaining of chest pain?
    a. 81 mg
    b. 324 mg
    c. 325 mg
    d. 162 mg - 325 mg

2. A patient experiencing chest pain with a history of coronary artery stent placement is most likely suffering from what?
    a. Acute stroke
    b. Acute coronary syndrome
    c. Tension pneumothorax
    d. Gallstones

3. Identify this rhythm.

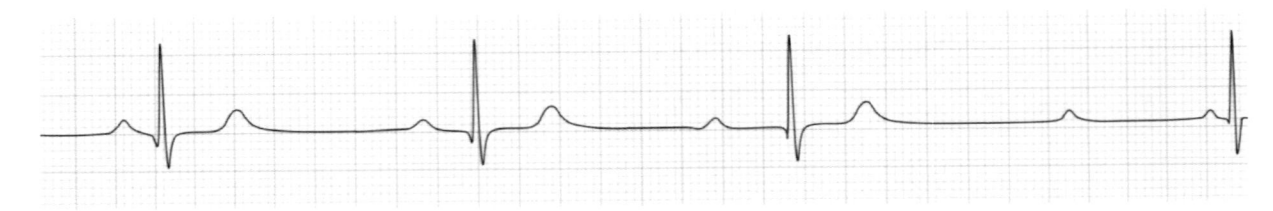

    a. Sinus bradycardia
    b. Second degree AV block type I
    c. Second degree AV block type II
    d. Third degree AV block

4. A patient in the emergency department waiting room collapses and remains unconscious, what is the next appropriate step a rescuer should take?
    a. Acquire a 12-lead ECG
    b. Perform a BLS assessment
    c. Begin CPR
    d. Provide rescue breaths

5.) Placement of an advanced airway should be confirmed by way of method?

   a. Chest x-ray

   b. Arterial blood gas

   c. Continuous waveform capnography

   d. Positive pressure ventilations

The following scenario applies to questions 6-10

Scenario: A 59-year-old man is being treated for chest pain and he appears diaphoretic, in obvious discomfort, and lightheaded. He has no prior medical history of cardiovascular disease. The 12-lead ECG reveals the rhythm below, which suddenly converts to ventricular fibrillation.

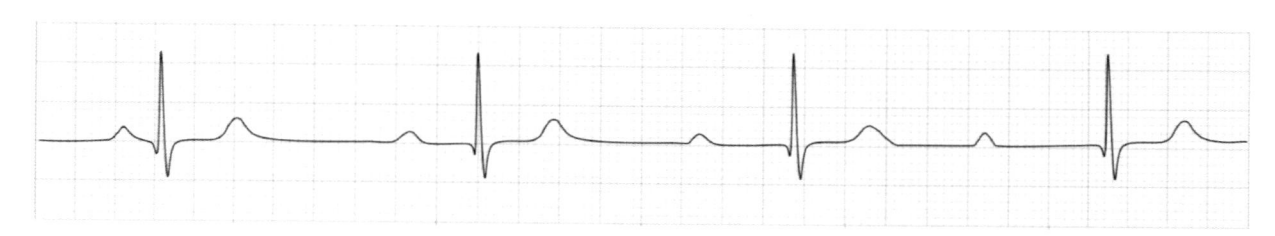

6. Identify the above rhythm.

   a. Wolff-Parkinson-White syndrome

   b. First degree AV block

   c. Second degree AV block type II

   d. Third degree AV block

7. What is the next most appropriate action to care for this patient?

   a. Place an advanced airway

   b. Perform defibrillation

   c. Perform synchronized cardioversion

   d. Perform transcutaneous pacing

8. Which medication should be administered first per the algorithm?

   a. Dopamine 2 mcg - 10 mcg/min

   b. Adenosine 12 mg

   c. Epinephrine 1 mg

   d. Amiodarone 300 mg

9. Despite the medication provided above the patient remains in ventricular fibrillation. Which medication should be provided next?

    a. Amiodarone 300 mg

    b. Epinephrine 1 mg

    c. Magnesium Sulfate 4 gm

    d. Epinephrine 2 mcg - 10 mcg/min

10. If the patient had not gone into ventricular fibrillation, what would have been the appropriate treatment?

    a. Synchronized cardioversion

    b. Vagal maneuvers

    c. Transcutaneous pacing

    d. Defibrillation

11. You are transporting a suspected stroke patient, what course of action takes priority upon arrival to the medical facility?

    a. Fibrinolytic therapy

    b. 12-lead ECG

    c. Pericardiocentesis

    d. CT scan

12. Patients suspected of having an acute coronary syndrome should be taken to which type of facility?

    a. Coronary reperfusion-capable facility

    b. Dialysis-capable facility

    c. A stroke center

    d. A level III trauma center

13. You are treating a suspected stroke patient who has a normal CT scan and has been experiencing symptoms for the last five hours, what is the next step in treatment?

    a. Request an MRI to confirm the CT scan

    b. Administer Fibrinolytic Therapy Immediately

    c. Refer patient for mechanical thrombectomy

    d. The patient requires no interventions

14. You are treating a patient with the below rhythm and is pulseless, what is the appropriate treatment?

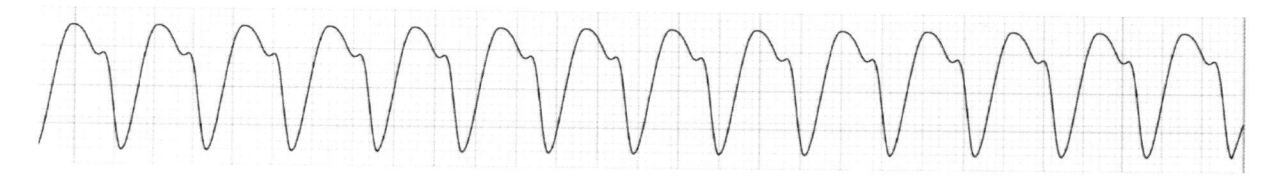

   a. Perform synchronized cardioversion
   b. Administer adenosine 6 mg
   c. Administer epinephrine 1 mg
   d. Perform defibrillation

15. Which action should immediately follow a defibrillation attempt?
   a. High-quality CPR
   b. Pulse/rhythm check
   c. Medication administration
   d. Another defibrillation if first attempt failed to resolve the rhythm

16. You notice a colleague performing shallow chest compressions, how should you address this?
   a. Wait until the end of the resuscitation
   b. Immediately take over chest compressions
   c. Say, "your compressions are wrong."
   d. Say, "ensure your compressions are 2 inches deep allowing for recoil."

17. The monitor displays a PETCO2 reading of 6 mmHg, what does this indicate?
   a. The patient is being hyperventilated
   b. Chest compressions are ineffective
   c. The patient is being hypoventilated
   d. The patient is developing a tension pneumothorax

18. You enter your patient's room, and they appear to be unconscious, but you hear them gasping, what action should be performed?
   a. Check the pulse oximeter reading
   b. Begin high-quality CPR the gasping is not normal breathing
   c. The gasping is normal breathing, and the patient does not require care
   d. Check the patient's blood glucose

19. Identify this rhythm

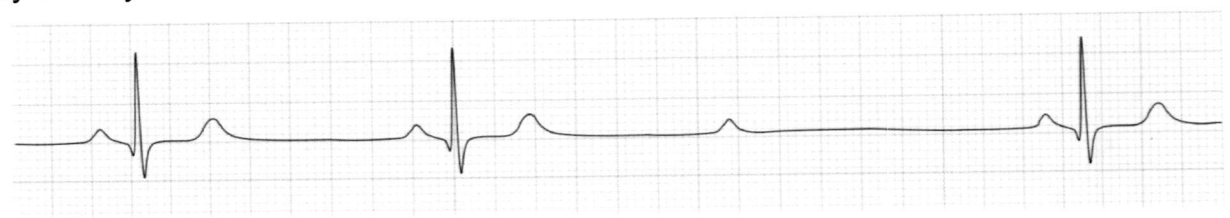

   a. First degree AV block
   b. Second degree AV block Type I
   c. Second degree AV block Type II
   d. Third degree AV block

20. You are treating a patient who just achieved ROSC but is unable to follow your commands, what treatment should be considered?
   a. 2 L fluid bolus
   b. Targeted temperature management
   c. Administer epinephrine 5 mcg/min drip
   d. Provide positive pressure ventilation 1 breath every 10 seconds

21. How is an OPA properly measured?
   a. From the corner of the nose to the earlobe
   b. From the corner of the mouth to the Adam's apple
   c. From the corner of the mouth to the corner of the jaw
   d. Sizes are universal, and measurement is not required

22. Targeted temperature management is provided at what temperature range?
   a. 30°C-34°C
   b. 31°C-35°C
   c. 32°C-36°C
   d. 33°C-37°C

23. How long should targeted temperature management be administered?
   a. 12 hours
   b. 24 hours
   c. 36 hours
   d. 48 hours

24. Increase chest compression fraction by performing what actions?
    a. Administer breaths while chest compressions are ongoing
    b. Administer medications while chest compressions are ongoing
    c. Switch compressors every two minutes
    d. Charge the defibrillator prior to the 2-minute mark

25. What reading provides insight into compression effectiveness?
    a. A palpable femoral pulse
    b. PETCO2 reading of at least 10 mmHg
    c. Pulse oxygen saturation
    d. Core body temperature

26. What is the purpose of having a CPR Coach?
    a. Ensure high-quality CPR is being performed
    b. Facilitate knowledge sharing
    c. To tell the team leader when he/she is wrong
    d. To perform defibrillation

27. What is the first medical intervention to balloon time for a STEMI patient?
    a. 30 minutes
    b. 60 minutes
    c. 90 minutes
    d. 120 minutes

28. What is the proper closed loop response for an order of amiodarone 300 mg?
    a. "Ok, got it.'
    b. "I have an order for amiodarone 300 mg."
    c. "Is that really what you want to give?"
    d. "I don't think that is correct."

29. How often should a breath be provided while performing rescue breaths?
    a. 1 breath every 2-3 seconds
    b. 1 breath every 5 seconds
    c. 1 breath every 6 seconds
    d. 1 breath every 10 seconds

30. A patient with a pulse and hypotension presents with the below rhythm, what action should be performed?

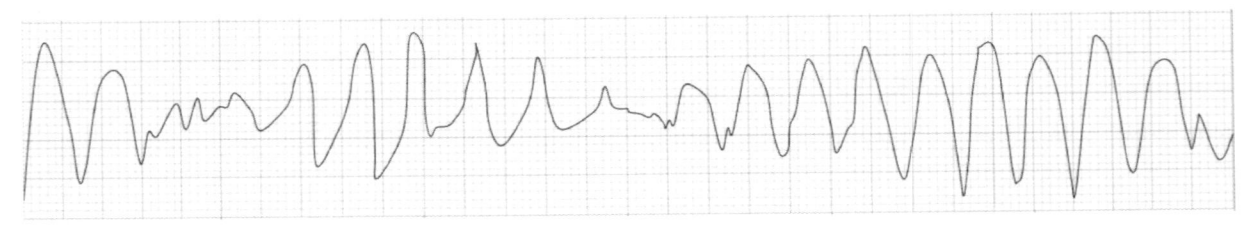

   a. Defibrillation
   b. Synchronized cardioversion
   c. Amiodarone 150 mg
   d. Dopamine 5 mg - 20 mg/kg/min infusion

31. Avoid excessive ventilation because it causes what?
   a. Optimal oxygenation
   b. Diminished cardiac output
   c. Improved circulation
   d. Decreased thoracic pressures

The following scenario applies to questions 32-40

Scenario: A 71-year-old patient was brought into the emergency department complaining of chest tightness, nausea, and dizziness. He explains that he had a heart attack two years ago.

32. What is the first and most important action to be taken?
   a. 12-lead ECG
   b. Cardiac panel
   c. ABG
   d. Blood glucose

33. The monitor reveals the below rhythm, identify this rhythm.

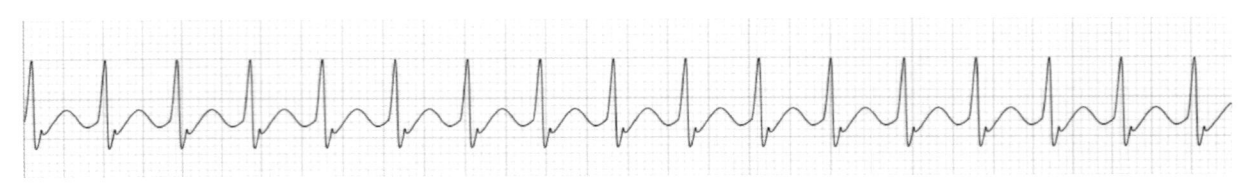

a. Atrial fibrillation

b. Atrial flutter

c. Sinus tachycardia

d. Supraventricular tachycardia

34. Given the patient's presentation and the above rhythm, what algorithm would be used to treat this patient?

    a. Cardiac arrest VF/pVT

    b. Adult tachycardia with a pulse

    c. Bradycardia

    d. Cardiac arrest PEA/Asystole

35. The patient's blood pressure is 84/68 mmHg. What is the most appropriate treatment for this patient?

    a. Vagal maneuvers

    b. Adenosine 6 mg

    c. Adenosine 12 mg

    d. Synchronized cardioversion

36. Despite the action above the patient's rhythm remains the same and the patient remains conscious. What is the next appropriate treatment?

    a. Vagal maneuvers

    b. Adenosine 6 mg

    c. Adenosine 12 mg

    d. Synchronized cardioversion

37. The patient goes unconscious, and the below rhythm presents on the monitor. What algorithm should the patient be treated under?

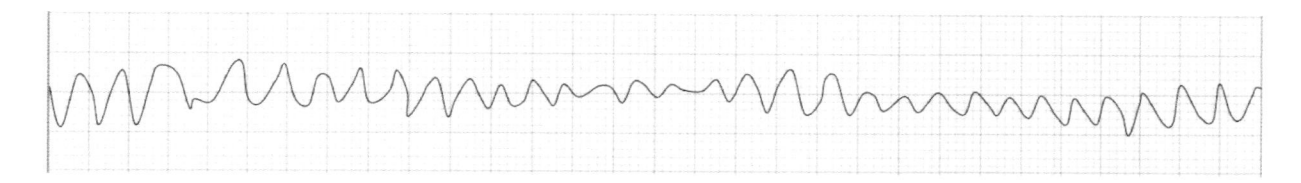

a. Cardiac arrest VF/pVT

b. Adult tachycardia with a pulse

c. Bradycardia

d. Cardiac arrest PEA/Asystole

38. Despite 2 defibrillation attempts, and epinephrine 1 mg the patient's condition does not improve. What medication should be given following the next defibrillation attempt?

   a. Lidocaine 1.5 mg IV push

   b. Atropine 1 mg IV push

   c. Beta blocker

   d. Adenosine 300 mg

39. The patient has a ROSC and remains unconscious. What should his minimum systolic blood pressure be?

   a. 80 mmHg

   b. 90 mmHg

   c. 94 mmHg

   d. 100 mmHg

40. Due to your patient being unconscious and unable to maintain an adequate ventilatory rate, what action takes priority?

   a. Lab values

   b. Chest x-ray

   c. Oxygen administration

   d. Advanced airway management

41. For a suspected stroke patient to receive fibrinolytic therapy they must have a symptom onset to needle time of what?

   a. 1 hour

   b. 1.5 hours

   c. 2 hours

   d. 3 hours

42. Which symptom indicates cardiac arrest
    a. Agonal gasps
    b. Erythema
    c. Ecchymosis
    d. Weak and thready pulse

43. If you notice that the team leader is becoming fixated on a particular course of action or therapy, what high-performance team dynamic should be utilized?
    a. Constructive intervention
    b. Knowledge sharing
    c. Establishing clear roles and responsibilities
    d. Identifying limitations

44. You are caring for a patient whose oxygen saturation is 88% on room air, what is an indicated treatment?
    a. Oxygen via non-rebreather mask
    b. Positive pressure ventilation
    c. Patient positioning
    d. Advanced airway management

45. Your patient complained of a fluttering feeling in their chest but denies any past medical history of cardiovascular disease. The below rhythm is seen on the monitor, your patient's blood pressure is 100/84, and does not appear to be in distress. What should your first course of action be?

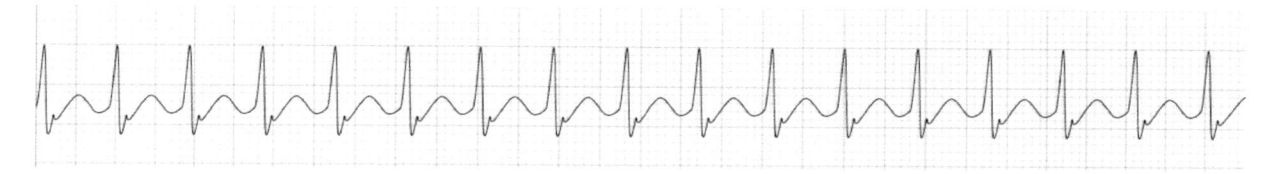

    a. Expert consultation
    b. Adenosine 6 mg
    c. Synchronized cardioversion
    d. Vagal maneuvers

46. What is the purpose of Medical Emergency Teams (MET) and Rapid Response Teams (RRT)?

   a. Provide guidance to resuscitation teams

   b. Improve patient outcomes by identifying clinical deterioration early

   c. Augment surgical teams in the event the patient enters cardiac arrest

   d. Facilitate patient transfers between EMS and the receiving hospital

47. A 53-year-old male is receiving chest compressions and at the two-minute mark remains pulseless, but this rhythm appears on the monitor. What should occur next?

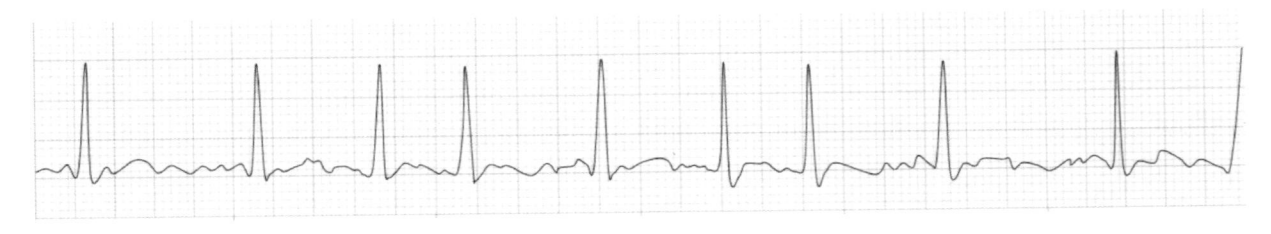

   a. The patient is in ROSC check responsiveness

   b. Perform synchronized cardioversion

   c. Resume CPR

   d. Perform defibrillation

48. Pauses in compressions should take no more than how long?

   a. 5 seconds

   b. 7 seconds

   c. 10 seconds

   d. 15 seconds

49. How long should a pulse and breathing check take?

   a. 1-2 seconds

   b. 3-6 seconds

   c. 5 seconds

   d. 5-10 seconds

50. What is the correct chest compression rate?

   a. 80/minute

   b. 100/minute

   c. 120/minute

   d. 100-120/minute

Conclusion

This brief resource covered the main criteria for mastering the ACLS discipline. Your understanding of the systematic approach, BLS criteria, the cardiovascular system, ECG interpretation skills, ACLS algorithms, airway management skills, and high-performance team dynamics is hopefully expanded. The AHA ACLS provider course assesses competency through completion of a 50-question written examination (passing score of 84%), and skills testing covering adult BLS, airway management, and a high-performance team activity involving a megacode. Megacode assessments will either start with a bradycardia or a tachycardia scenario and degrade into cardiac arrest VF/pVT, PEA/Asystole and finally ROSC. Understand that emergency cardiovascular care is dynamic. Advances in treatment occur rapidly, check for changes in recommended drugs and respective doses here www.heart.org/courseupdates. Visit EMskillz.com to see our current and upcoming products. Thank you for your dedication to emergency medicine and for ensuring the highest quality patient care available.

References

ECG - Knowledge @ amboss. ambossIcon. (2021, September 21). Retrieved November 19, 2021, from https://www.amboss.com/us/knowledge/ECG/.

Heward SJ, Widrich J. Coronary Perfusion Pressure. [Updated 2020 Jul 10]. In: StatPearls [Internet]. Treasure Island (FL): StatPearls Publishing; 2021 Jan-. Available from: https://www.ncbi.nlm.nih.gov/books/NBK551531/

Sinz, E., Navarro, K., Cheng, A., & Hunt, E. A. (2020). Advanced cardiovascular life support: provider manual. American Heart Association.

Torsades de pointes: Treatment, symptoms, and causes, https://www.medicalnewstoday.com/articles/320619.

Pretest/Posttest Answer Keys

1) D	26) A
2) B	27) C
3) B	28) B
4) B	29) C
5) C	30) B
6) D	31) B
7) B	32) A
8) C	33) D
9) A	34) B
10) C	35) A
11) D	36) B
12) A	37) A
13) C	38) A
14) D	39) B
15) A	40) D
16) D	41) D
17) B	42) A
18) B	43) B
19) C	44) A
20) B	45) D
21) C	46) B
22) C	47) C
23) B	48) C
24) D	49) D
25) B	50) D

Checks on Learning Answers

Page 19

> ✓
> - What assessment is used for an unconscious patient?
> - What does SAMPLE stand for?
> - Reversible causes are also known as what?
> - Name 3 reversible causes.
> - Which questions quickly allow you to assess a patient's status?

- BLS Assessment
- Signs and Symptoms, Allergies, Medications, Past medical history, Last oral intake, Events
- Hs & Ts
- Hypoxia, Hypovolemia, Hypothermia, Hypokalemia, Hyperkalemia, Hydrogen ion acidosis, Thrombus coronary, Thrombus pulmonary, Tamponade cardiac, Tension Pneumothorax, Toxins
- Is a pulse present?, What is the heart rate?, Is the patient stable or unstable?

Page 22

> ✓
> - How long should pauses in compressions be kept to?
> - What is the required chest compression rate?
> - What is the adult compression depth?
> - PETCO2/ETCO2 of 10 mmHg indicates what?
> - Perform what action at the 1:45 minute mark to maximize CCF?

- 10 seconds
- 100-120 compressions per minute
- 2 inches
- Effective chest compressions
- Charge the defibrillator

Page 28

> - Where does a sinus rhythm originate?
> - One small block equals how many seconds?
> - One large block equals how many seconds?
> - What is the normal adult heart rate?

- The SA node
- 0.04 seconds
- 0.2 seconds
- 60-100 beats per minute

Page 31

> - Which 'A' named medications belong to the following algorithms:
>   - Cardiac Arrest
>   - Tachycardia
>   - Bradycardia
> - What is the first and second dose of amiodarone?
> - Epinephrine administration is spaced out by how many minutes?

- Cardiac Arrest – amiodarone
- Tachycardia – adenosine
- Bradycardia – atropine
- 300 mg, 150 mg
- 3-5 minutes

Page 35

> - Which medication follows the second defibrillation attempt?
> - What action immediately follows defibrillation/pulse and rhythm check?
> - What action increases CCF?
> - A patient in VF requires what treatment?
> - Which medication is an alternative to amiodarone?

- 1 mg epinephrine
- Resumption of chest compressions
- Charging the defibrillator
- Defibrillation
- Lidocaine, first dose 1.0-1.5 mg/kg, second dose 0.5-0.75 mg/kg

Page 39

> - What heart rate indicates bradycardia?
> - Which AV block has a consistent PR-interval > 0.2 seconds?
> - Which AV block has a PR-interval that increases until the QRS complex falls off?
> - What AV block looks normal except random QRS complexes drop-off?
> - Which AV block has consistent P:P and R:R intervals but has no relation between the P-waves and QRS complexes?

- < 60 beats per minute
- First degree
- Second degree type I
- Second degree type II
- Third degree

Page 42

> - Tachyarrhythmias are over how many beats per minute?
> - SVT exceeds what heart rate?
> - What is a uniformly shaped VT called?

- 100 beats per minute
- 150 beats per minute
- Monomorphic Ventricular Tachycardia

Page 47

> ✓
> - Can an OPA be used to manage a conscious patient's airway?
> - How is an OPA measured?
> - What PETCO2 reading must be maintained to indicate effective compressions?
> - What is used to confirm endotracheal tube placement?
> - What is the normal PETCO2 range?

- No
- From the corner of the mouth to the corner of the jaw
- 10 mmHg
- Continuous waveform capnography
- 35-45 mmHg

Page 50

> ✓
> - What is the purpose of METs and RRTs?
> - A team member unable to perform a task should do what?
> - Correcting a team member before they can make a mistake is known as what?
> - High-performance teams utilize what type of communication?
> - What is the CPR Coach's purpose?

- Identify and treat early clinical deterioration to optimize patient outcomes
- Request a new role
- Constructive Intervention
- Closed-loop communication
- Ensure high-quality CPR is always conducted

ECG ANALYSIS TOOL

5 Step ECG Analysis

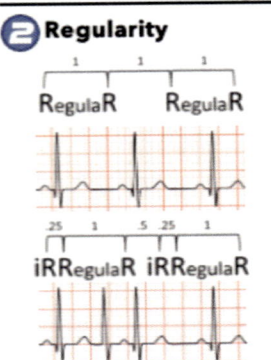

② Regularity

③ P waves

Present? Rounded and ≤ 2.5 mm? If not, impulse may not originate from SA node. Multiple P waves can be the result of PACs or AV Block

④ QRS complex

> 3 mm (0.12 s) = Wide QRS / missing QRS(s) may indicate AV Block

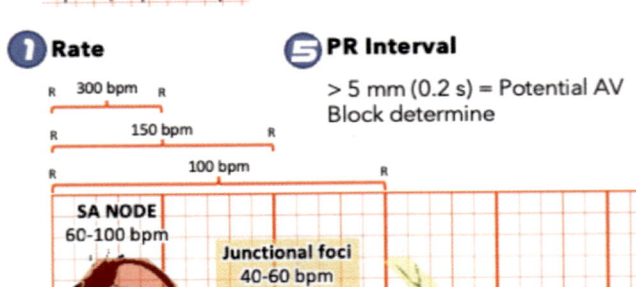

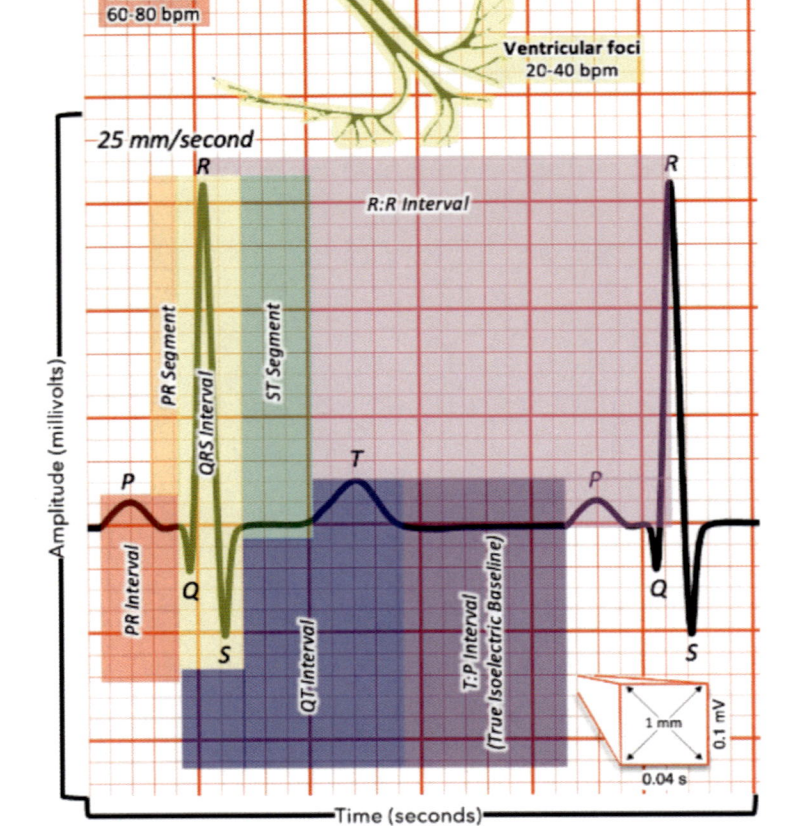

① Rate

⑤ PR Interval

> 5 mm (0.2 s) = Potential AV Block determine

- SA NODE 60-100 bpm
- Junctional foci 40-60 bpm
- Atrial foci 60-80 bpm
- Ventricular foci 20-40 bpm

25 mm/second

PAILS Method

Region	Leads	Vessel	Treatment
Posterior	V1-V4	LCX	MONA
Anterior	V2-V4	LAD	MONA
Inferior	II, III, aVF	RCA	2L Fluid bolus, no nitro, no β Blockers
Lateral	I, aVL, V5, V6	LCX	MONA
Septal	V1, V2	LAD	MONA

12-lead Placement

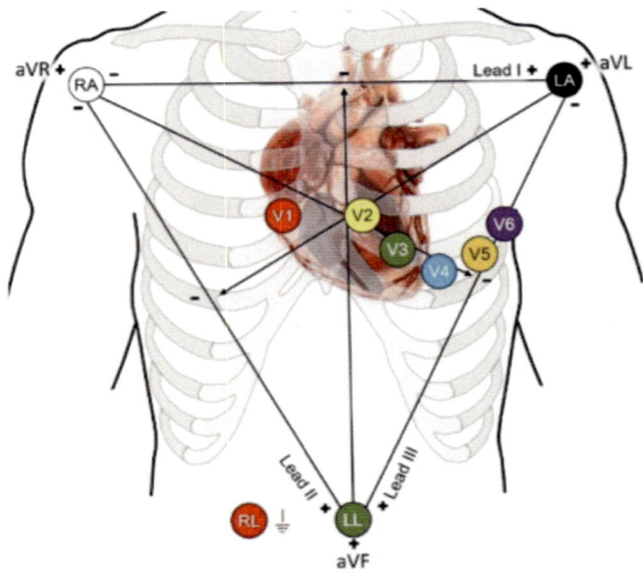

Normal Sinus Rhythm Parameters
viewed from lead II

Heart Rate:	60-100/min
P wave:	Atrial depolarization Amplitude: ≤ 2.5 mm Duration: < 0.12 s
PR Segment:	AV node depolarization, baseline for measuring ST elevation
PR Interval:	Time electricity takes to move through the atrium and the atrioventricular junction Duration: 0.12 s - 0.2 s
QRS interval:	Ventricular depolarization Duration: 0.06 s - 0.12 s **Q:** Ventricular septal depolarization **Amplitude:** ≤ 1/3 of R wave amplitude **R:** Apical ventricular depolarization **Amplitude:** ≤ 20 mm **S:** Basal ventricular depolarization
ST segment:	1 mm elevation in two contiguous leads other than V2, and V3 (2 mm).
T wave:	Ventricular repolarization **Amplitude:** 6 mm
QT interval:	QT ≤ 0.40 s @ 70 bpm; for every 10 bpm ↑ 70 subtract 0.02 s, and for every 10 bpm ↓ 70 add 0.02 sec

EMERGENCY CARDIOVASCULAR CARE DATA SHEET

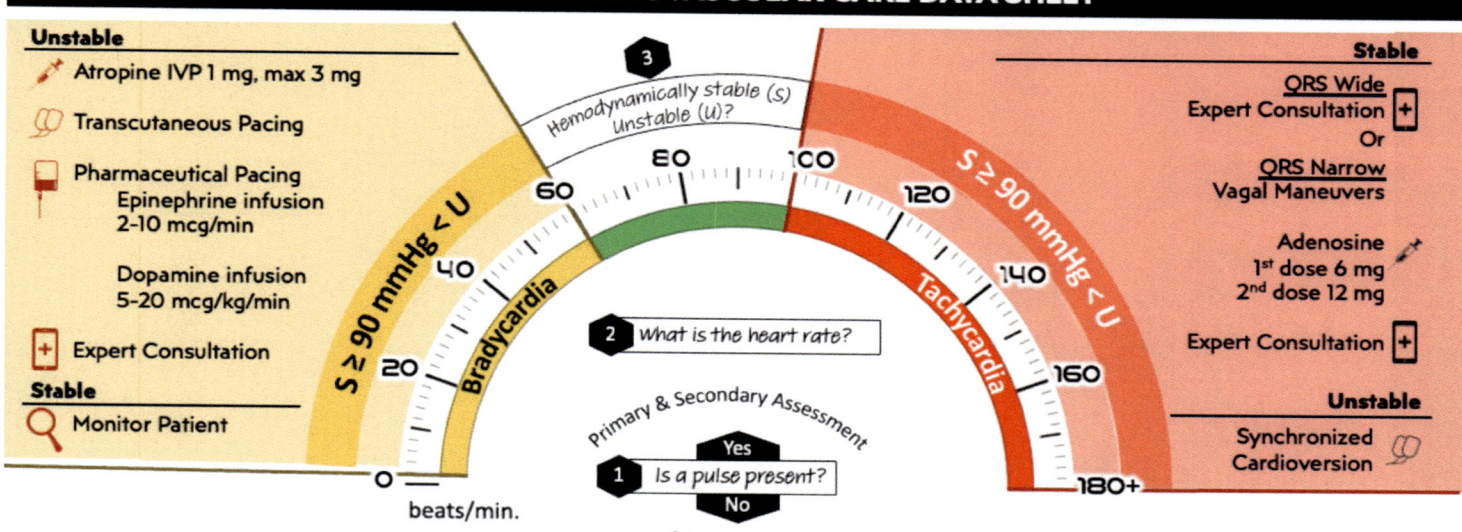

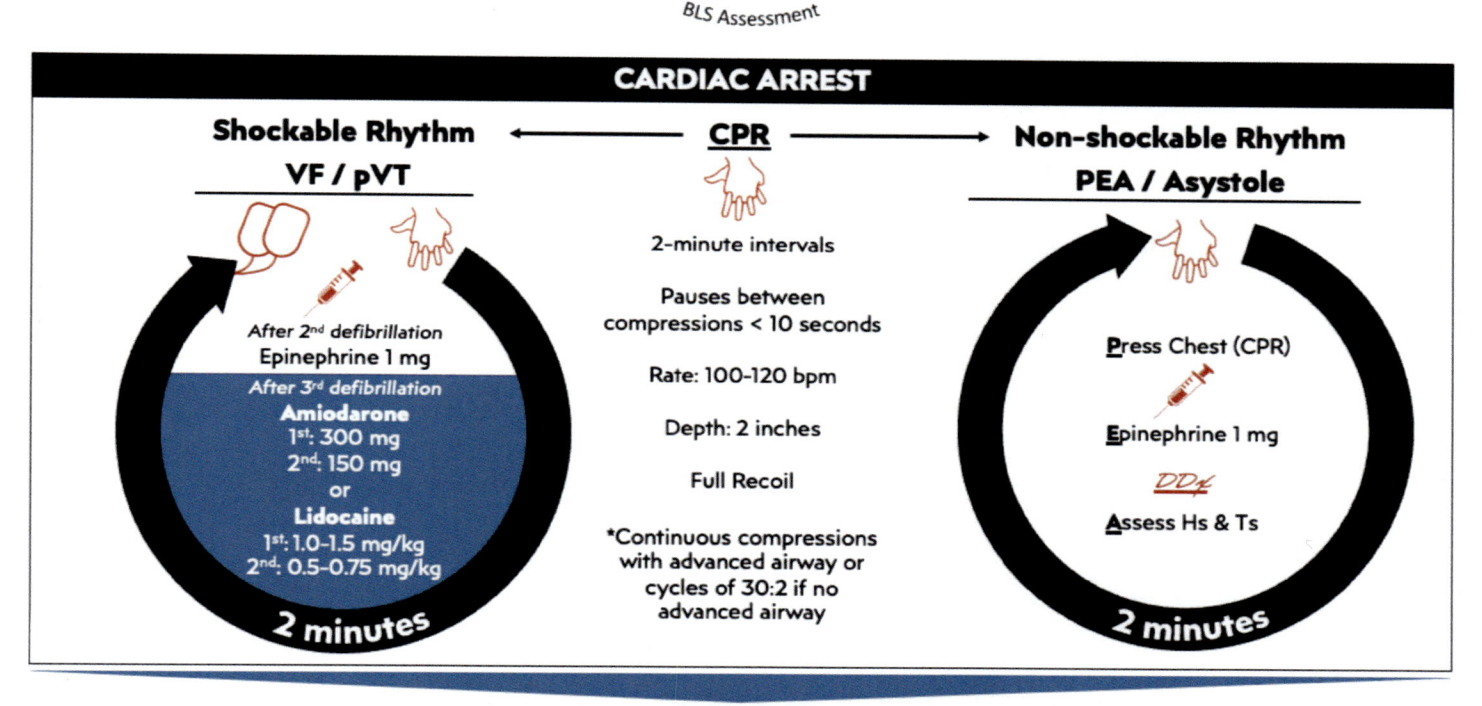

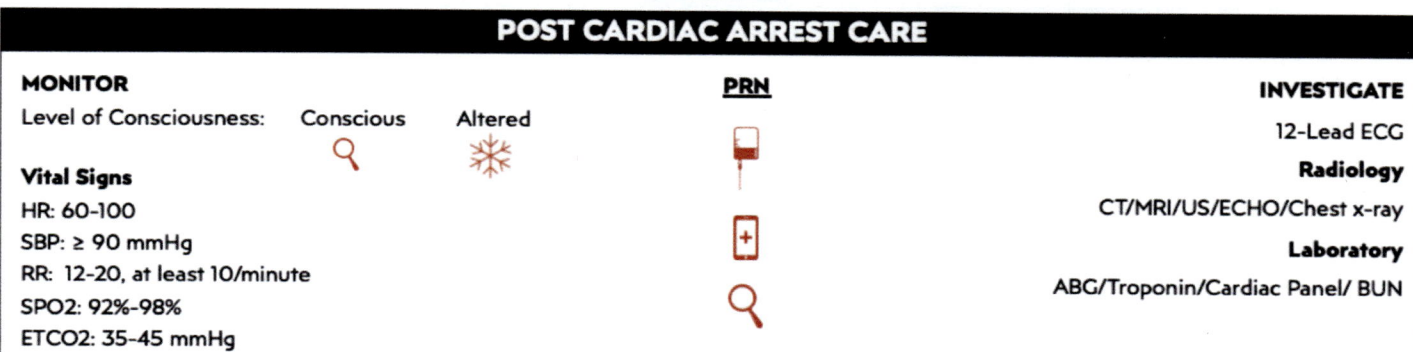

Unstable
- Atropine IVP 1 mg, max 3 mg
- Transcutaneous Pacing
- Pharmaceutical Pacing
  Epinephrine infusion
  2-10 mcg/min
  Dopamine infusion
  5-20 mcg/kg/min
- Expert Consultation

Stable
- Monitor Patient

Stable
- QRS Wide
  Expert Consultation
  Or
- QRS Narrow
  Vagal Maneuvers
  Adenosine
  1st dose 6 mg
  2nd dose 12 mg
  Expert Consultation

Unstable
- Synchronized Cardioversion

3. Hemodynamically stable (S) Unstable (U)?
2. What is the heart rate?
1. Is a pulse present? — Yes → Primary & Secondary Assessment / No → BLS Assessment

Bradycardia: S ≥ 90 mmHg < U (0–60 beats/min)
Tachycardia: S ≥ 90 mmHg < U (100–180+ beats/min)

CARDIAC ARREST

Shockable Rhythm ← CPR → **Non-shockable Rhythm**
VF / pVT   PEA / Asystole

Shockable (2 minutes):
After 2nd defibrillation
Epinephrine 1 mg
After 3rd defibrillation
Amiodarone
1st: 300 mg
2nd: 150 mg
or
Lidocaine
1st: 1.0-1.5 mg/kg
2nd: 0.5-0.75 mg/kg

CPR:
- 2-minute intervals
- Pauses between compressions < 10 seconds
- Rate: 100-120 bpm
- Depth: 2 inches
- Full Recoil
- *Continuous compressions with advanced airway or cycles of 30:2 if no advanced airway

Non-shockable (2 minutes):
- Press Chest (CPR)
- Epinephrine 1 mg
- DDx
- Assess Hs & Ts

POST CARDIAC ARREST CARE

MONITOR
Level of Consciousness: Conscious   Altered

Vital Signs
HR: 60-100
SBP: ≥ 90 mmHg
RR: 12-20, at least 10/minute
SPO2: 92%-98%
ETCO2: 35-45 mmHg

PRN

INVESTIGATE
12-Lead ECG
Radiology
CT/MRI/US/ECHO/Chest x-ray
Laboratory
ABG/Troponin/Cardiac Panel/ BUN

ICON LEGEND

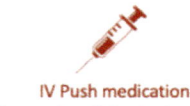

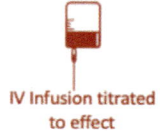

- IV Push medication — Doses given 3-5 minutes apart
- CPR
- Bradycardia: Transcutaneous Pacing / Tachycardia: Sync. Cardioversion 100J-150J / Cardiac Arrest: Defibrillation 150J-200J
- IV Infusion titrated to effect
- Expert Consultation
- Targeted Temp Mgmt. 32 C-36 C x 24 hrs. + EEG
- Monitor Patient

Made in the USA
Monee, IL
27 October 2023